The Miles

and Trials

of a

Marathon

Goddess

52 Weeks, 52 Marathons:
The Miles and Trials
of a Marathon Goddess

Copyright © Julie Weiss 2019

Quantity Sales availalbe.
For details contact the author at the email address above.

Printed in the United States of America

ISBN: 978-1-7326927-2-5
The Miles and Trials of a Marathon Goddess
Author: Julie Weiss with Ali Nolan and John Hanc
All rights reserved

Library of Congress
ID: 1-7370674941
January 2019
101 Independence Avenue
Washington, DC 20559-6000

The events described in this book are the real experiences of real people. However, in a number of cases, the authors have changed names and disguised identities to respect privacy.

52 Weeks, 52 Marathons:

The Miles and Trials

of a Marathon Goddess

By Julie Weiss

With Ali Nolan and John Hanc

Dear Omi ♡ We Got This! Love Julie Weiss xo, Marathon Goddess . ! Heres to the cure! ♡

Tender Fire Books/Enhanced Communications, LLC 2019

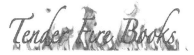

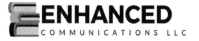

To Papa.

And in memory of Lupe.

The Miles and Trials of a Marathon Goddess

Table of Contents

FOREWORD

The most amazing thing about running is how it transforms us as a whole — How we can move from withdrawn to confident, tentative to deliberate — the list goes on and on, and the stories about these transformations are endlessly fascinating.

Julie Weiss was a self-proclaimed bad girl, an in-your-face teenager and out-of-control single mom who transformed herself through running into a beautiful woman who ran many thoughtful miles, found her own identity and took charge of her destiny. That included restoring a love with her estranged father. She became like the mythical goddess emerging from the tumult of the sea.

But running is about more than transformation; it can give redemption and resolution. Nobody can run and stay angry, and nobody can run with a broken heart without eventually finding healing.

Not long after their reconciliation, Julie's father suddenly died. No sooner did she have him back than she lost him again forever. The bigger story here is not about Julie, but how the Goddess emerged from her to make her father live on endlessly.

Kathrine Switzer, first woman to officially enter and run the Boston Marathon; author, Marathon Woman; and founder of 261 Fearless (www.261fearless.org), a global community of women runners.

INTRODUCTION

Being a goddess isn't all it's cracked up to be.

That's what I'm thinking as I stare into my bathroom mirror, early on the morning of Sunday, March 19, 2017. And when I say early, I mean it is practically last night: A little after 3 a.m., when I dragged myself out of my bed after five sleepless hours.

I stare at my puffy, bloodshot eyes, my bed-head hair, and wonder why.

Why am I about to run the City of Los Angeles Marathon, two days after having to dose myself with a Z-Pak of antibiotics to ward off the flu?

Why am I about to travel 26.2 miles on my already-aching feet just one day before I'm scheduled to board a flight to Paris with my mom to visit my daughter and grandchild?

Perhaps most damning: Why am I about to run my 104th career marathon on very little training?

Good questions. Yet, the answer, even at this hour, is as obvious and bracing as the Pacific Ocean breeze wafting through my apartment window: Because I have to.

My name is Julie Weiss, and although I call myself The Marathon Goddess, I certainly don't claim any divine powers, unless you count tenacity as a gift from above. And that tenaciousness—okay, my husband might have a few different words to describe it—is what drives the story of my unlikely route to some prominence in the world of marathon running and fund raising. I have been honored to have my story told on The Today Show, CNN and ESPN; in a popular documentary film, *Spirit of the Marathon II*; as well as publications from O Magazine to the Los Angeles Times.

My claim to fame is having done something that, even in our marathon-mad culture, only two or three others have achieved: In 2012-13, I ran 52 marathons in 52 weeks. I did it to help raise money to fight pancreatic cancer, the insidious disease that claimed the life of my father Maurice Weiss, with whom I had a tumultuous relationship during my very troubled youth. But my running, which I began at a low point in my life, had brought us back together. Then, right before I qualified for my first Boston marathon, he was diagnosed with the disease. He was gone 35 days later.

That crazy 52/52 streak—something only a few others had done at the time—was my tribute to him; and he is a big part of my story.

Those races in my year-long marathon streak were run everywhere from the ancient streets of Rome, Italy—where *Spirit of the Marathon* was filmed—to the mysterious corridors of Area 51, over the course of a jet-lagged year that felt like I was caught in a vortex of boarding passes, Power Bars and the safety pins used to fasten the race bibs to my singlet. On and off those race numbers flew, like the calendar pages in an old movie, flipping through to show the passage of time, as I ran my way around the country, 26.2 miles at a clip, following an itinerary that would fatigue an airline crew:

Miami, Denver, Austin, Phoenix, Seattle, Boston.

I was indefatigable in my pursuit of the 52-week goal: Neither a full time job, Superstorm Sandy or a case of chronic jet lag that even Starbucks was unable to cure could stop me.

I started and finished my year-long marathon odyssey right here.

I'm a SoCal girl, born and raised in Santa Monica. So

much so I never wanted to even go east of the 405, the north-south interstate that bisects Los Angeles and is legendary for its Armageddon traffic jams. My Left Coast upbringing is an important part of my story. In fact, let me amend slightly that description of a few sentences earlier. I was a SoCal bad girl. Very bad. Hung with the wrong crowd, did things I shouldn't have (some of them fun, others not).

I was pregnant with my son at age 17; had my daughter when I was 22. (Frankie and Samantha are now 30 and 25 years old, respectively). When their father and I split up, I went through a long period of depression, probably because I realized how badly I had already screwed up my life. There I was, a too-young single mom, a high school drop-out, a kid raising kids. Over the next decade, I gained weight and wallowed in self-pity as I struggled to make it as a single mom. Eventually, I sought help and was given drugs, which made it worse. Finally, at age 37, I hit bottom: I was 35 pounds overweight, and my emotional trough ran so deep that antidepressants weren't enough: I was given extra-strength antidepressants. Up the dosage! That was the psychiatric community's answer for me.

Fortunately, I found a better alternative: Hawaii. Who wouldn't feel better in the Aloha State? Me. At least initially.

During my family's 2007 vacation on Hanalei Beach, I felt like a beached whale. The relationship with my father, Maurice Weiss, didn't help. We called him Papa, and he fit the part. A bear of a man, with a rakish white van dyke and a ready smile, he could, when he wanted to, be quite charming. He didn't want to with me—at least not at that point in our lives. At the time of the Hawaii vacation we were barely on speaking terms. Which might have been an improvement over what he had been saying when we were speaking. "You're fat" and "Get the fuck out of here!" were among the lovely comments he'd made to me in the previous few years.

My response to was to cry my eyes out and feel sorry for myself.

Don't get me wrong: I'm not excusing my dad's abusive language. It was wrong, it was insensitive. But Maurice Weiss was a Depression-era kid who had his own issues. As well as his own exotic backstory and claims to fame:

He was born in New York in 1935. His father, Sammy Weiss, was a prominent jazz drummer who played with some of the great Big Band leaders of that time, including Benny Goodman, Tommy Dorsey and Artie Shaw. Dad inherited some of his father's talent. He was a prodigy on the drums, and as a kid performed regularly on the NBC radio show "Coast to Coast on the Bus" with Milton Cross. He also played piano and trumpet. At some point during my dad's childhood, however, the Weiss family moved west, supposedly because of my father's asthma. It wasn't exactly a California Gold Rush for the Weiss family. While my grandfather continued to find work—he performed on the Jack Benny Show—the sense we got, from my parents and from my aunt and uncle, was that Sammy Weiss's career took a hit when he moved out here, and he took it out on his son. Whether there was physical abuse, we don't know. But my sister and I suspect that our dad carried a lot of Jewish guilt around for having had the nerve to be asthmatic and screw up his father's musical career.

And probably some anger, too.

Despite such misgivings and shortcomings, Maurice had gone on to a respectable if conventional career as a stockbroker. And while the kind and funny Papa I remembered as a little girl wasn't winning Father of the Year awards by the time he was in late middle age, he did manage to reinvent himself yet again. He cancelled his Wall Street Journal subscription for a life of Variety. At age 70, Maurice Weiss found a new career as an actor. He did a few independent movies and then landed a Sprint commercial. Some other commercial work followed, including a bizarre and probably little-seen ad for a Japanese camera in which my dad howled like a dog.

Strange, but very cool.

Now, I was ready to howl, too. But I wasn't acting: I desperately needed a new life. On the beach one morning during that Hawaii vacation, I took the first tentative steps in search of it. I'm not sure what compelled me that day to walk down by the shoreline and start running. I'd liked to run as a kid, but probably so did some of the kids who would grow up to become the stars of "My 600 Pound Life." Most children like to run around, but few of them come back to it as adults. In my case, I had bottomed out; I knew I had to do something, I was tired of the drugs, and sick and tired of feeling like shit. Running seemed the most direct and available route to a new me.

I jogged, walked and stumbled nearly a mile that day before I collapsed in the white sands, gasping for air. But something in me awoke. For the very first time in I don't remember how long, I began to feel alive again. It was if I was being reinvigorated by the energy of the sea, the waves and the sand. I felt great, like I had really accomplished something.

That very same night, I stopped taking my anti-depressants. I knew this was what I'd been looking for.

Granted, everything looks better on vacation—and especially when your holiday is in Paradise. As soon as I got back home from Hawaii, I took my four-year-old dog Jessie and headed out on the pristine sands of Santa Monica beach. I wanted to see if this running thing was for real. The first time, I couldn't even make it from one lifeguard tower to the next—just a few hundred feet. But with Jessie, a Chow-Golden Retriever mix, matching me stride for stride, I tried again and again. Soon, I was running the length of two towers... three... and then, miracle of miracles, I was able to complete a mile without stopping, without even walking!

When I ran something remarkable happened: I felt uplifted, proud, renewed and resurgent. Was it all some kind of chemically-induced runner's high, a brain-soothing cocktail of serotonin and cannabinoids that was responsible for this euphoric feeling? Who knows? Who cares? I was hooked. Instead of some of the losers I'd been partying with most of my life, I decided to seek out the company of those who were well entrenched in this new running culture. I found my groove, and many new friends, with the L.A. Road Runners, a large and well-established club of running devotees.

It was my dad who told me about the Road Runners. Yes, the old abusive cuss—which is how I viewed him at that point—

had been impressed by my attempts to start running and decided that pointing me in the direction of a local running club was more constructive than pointing out my flabby tush and zaftig thighs. I remember how surprised I was the night he called me to make that suggestion. The conversations at that point were still cool, but not hostile. I began to feel just a glimmer of the warmth and love that I had known from him as a child.

As far as the L.A. Road Runners, Dad was right. Running with a group helped me enormously. As it has for thousands of others. In April 2017, the *New York Times* reported on research suggesting that running may be socially contagious. In the study, runners who were part of a network of other runners were positively influenced by one another. If one person in the group ran about 10 minutes longer, their friends would lengthen their workout accordingly; if someone picked up the pace, others responded in kind. The study seemed to prove what runners have known for a long time: training with others is beneficial. The idea that running must be this grim, solitary labor is more than old school thinking; it's just not true. I learned that with the L.A. Road Runners, where I flourished in that large and well-established group. At first, I still felt like such a loser, and they all seemed so cool -- fit, confident, upbeat. But they were also welcoming and encouraging and after a while, I found that I was able to keep up in the training runs.

I joined the L.A. Road Runners in January, 2008. Just two months later, I completed my first marathon (the L. A. Marathon, where else?).

Yes, I was drawn into running, hook, line and sneaker. But along with new friends, a revived sense of confidence and self-worth, and a commitment to a healthy activity, I found something else of vital importance: a new relationship with my father.

Papa had successfully reinvented himself professionally. I think when he heard that I was now seriously trying to make a change, and a positive one, it warmed his heart. Sharp right turns in mid-life were something he understood. We began talking regularly on the phone. The conversations were supportive, not critical. He even came out to see me for that first marathon, and although we failed to find each other at the crowded finish line area that day, a profound reconnection had begun. Maurice became my biggest fan. He also enjoyed the whole running scene, and seeing him along the course of the races, cheering me on, made my spirits soar.

Papa also fanned my competitive flames. Growing up back East, he knew about the famous Boston Marathon. While completing any 26.2-mile race is an achievement, Boston is the only major marathon that demands entrants demonstrate a level of competence. You have to have already achieved a certain time at the marathon distance, based on your age and gender, in order to enter the race. My father began studying these qualifying times, and suggested to me that I should try and go for my "BQ"—Boston Qualifier. He kind of made it sound like only then could I truly call myself a runner.

I'd heard about Boston from some of my new friends in the Road Runners. Mid-pack runners like me, most of them dream of qualifying for the granddaddy of all marathons. But it seemed a daunting task to meet my qualifying standard, which at that point was 3 hours 50 minutes. Not that I couldn't go the distance. By then, I was starting to run a 26.2 mile race every couple of months. I had even gotten to the point that I was a pace leader for the Road Runners, meaning that I could lead a group of less experienced runners at a pre-determined pace and hold that, for mile after mile. Running steady and getting faster, however, are too different things. After every marathon, I'd call my father. His first question: "Did you do it? Did you qualify for Boston?" The old dad would have probably called me a failure when I'd told him no. But now, he'd buck me up. "Keep trying, Julie. You're going to do it one of these days, I know."

"Thanks, Papa," I'd reply. "I really appreciate your confidence in me."

No lie. I was so happy to have my dad back in my life; my new life as a svelte runner, who had lost 35 pounds in six months; a woman who felt good about herself for the first time in years. It looked like this was going to be a beautiful story of reconciliation: Estranged daughter becomes runner, makes father proud. They are then reunited in supportive, happy love for one another and the family lives together happily ever after.

But that's not the way it panned out. In October, my father was diagnosed with Stage 4 pancreatic cancer. Then, just as he and I and the rest of our family were wrapping our heads around this life-changing news—he was gone.

Maurice Weiss died November 24, 2010, 35 days after he was diagnosed.

Two weeks later, heartsick but determined, I ran 3:47.19 and qualified for my first Boston Marathon.

I felt as if for the second time in my life, I'd lost my father. But this time it was permanent. I decided to dedicate myself to helping fight the disease that had taken him away from me so suddenly, and that continues to kill so many others. Pancreatic cancer, I'd learned, is the third most lethal form of cancer in America, but one of the most underfunded. Maybe I could do something about that, I thought. But what would that be? I'm not a scientist or a researcher.

Then it hit me. My new passion that dad had so vigorously supported was the perfect vehicle to help fight the disease that had taken his life. I became part of the charity running movement, an enormous engine of change that has propelled the growth in marathon participation over the last two decades, while funneling many dollars into the coffers of many good causes.

As I have with many things in my life, I took this to the extreme: Not for me, a fund raising 5K here or there. Not even an annual marathon in which I'd raise money for a pancreatic cancer prevention charity.

No, for me, it had to be a marathon a week.

I'm not sure how or when I had the idea. At the time, I'd only heard of one guy who had done it, Dane Rauschenberg, a runner from Washington, D.C. who achieved his 52-in-52 in 2006.

Nobody else had done it that I knew of (and to this day, few have). I remember the morning I woke up and it popped in my head. I knew it was a crazy idea, I didn't know how I was going to do it, but darn it, I was going to do it. That same night I went on MarathonGuide.com and had my whole scheduled picked out in three hours.

During that Grand Tour of marathons, I became The Marathon Goddess. I originally saw it on a t-shirt and thought "That's cool." Quite honestly it seemed to give me permission to do what I like to do in a marathon: Have fun, encourage others, interact with the spectators. So as the Marathon Goddess, I started high-fiving, dancing and prancing my way through 26.2 miles from Napa Valley to New Orleans.

Let's face it: These big city marathons, in addition to being serious athletic events and monumental individual challenges, are also a form of street theater. Coming from a family of musicians and entertainers, I guess it's not a surprise that when I run, I like to put on a bit of a show—for my fellow runners, for the spectators, for the people who've supported our cause with donations. I can and will talk to anybody, and I have no problem cajoling perfect strangers to cheer, sing or dance, even while we're running. It's all positive, it's all fun, it's all for a good cause, whether that cause is self- actualization, competition, a shared activity with like-minded people or fundraising.

Although I'd never considered myself much of an athlete, my marathon antics—and fund raising—were attracting notice. When I crossed the finish line of race number 52 on March 17,

2013—in my hometown City of Los Angeles Marathon—I was surrounded by as many cameras as the winners.

The fund-raising continued well past 2013. I'm still at it. As of now, I've raised more than $500,000 for pancreatic cancer charities, most notably the L.A.-based Hirshberg Foundation for Pancreatic Cancer Research and the El Segundo-based Pancreatic Cancer Action Network— organizations that have become like an extended family for me. And I continue to run marathons (although not on a weekly basis!) My 100th was the 2016 City of Los Angeles Marathon. I achieved a singular honor that day—one usually reserved for athletes in the major sports making last-minute baskets or throwing game-winning touchdown passes—when a clip of me crossing the finish line of my 100th marathon was ESPN's "Play of the Day."

Now here I am in the pre-dawn darkness of a Sunday in March, 2017, back again, for my 104th marathon. Indeed, the very thought of it momentarily overwhelms me. Scrunching my face into a scowl, I arrive at what I think is a momentous decision.

"David," I call out to my husband, who is getting ready in the bedroom.

"Yes?"

"This is my last marathon."

"OK," he says.

Pause.

"Julie?"

"What?"

"We need to leave in about five minutes."

This is what I love about David. He knows how to handle the moods and whims of a Marathon Goddess.

###

If a homeless person drove a Lexus, it would be David's. A 2000 Lexus Rx300, it has about two million miles on its odometer, and its exterior is as weathered as the face of a pioneer in the Mojave desert, in part because David uses it less as a sports car and more like a pick-up truck, hauling supplies for the runners he coaches to their weekly training runs in Griffith Park.

It was quite a crowd packed into the Lexus that morning. There were 2,600 water cups, a 12 x 12 awning, a 10-gallon water cooler, a case of Gatorade, banners, two 6-foot tables—and me.

I sat in the back seat, grumpily checking my Facebook page. Even all the "Go, Julie!" messages of support from my friends and followers weren't cheering me up at that moment. David whistled a happy tune in the front. Hmmm... I wonder. David knew I was in a bad mood. Did he really need 2,600 cups or was that just a way to conveniently stash me in the back? A shrewd man, my hubby! And I don't blame him. I am still cranky as I glared out at Los Angeles shrouded in darkness.

"Yeah, this is definitely my last marathon."

"Okay," says David matter-of-factly from the front.

It's 4:30 a.m. when David turns his car down the access road into the shallow canyon known as Chavez Ravine, site of Dodger Stadium and the start of the City of Los Angeles Marathon. This is the 32nd annual edition of the race that once was confined mostly to the inner city, but now sweeps west in a veritable tour of LA-LA Land, from the Stadium through Hollywood, Beverly Hills, Century City, Westwood, Brentwood and, finally, to the finish in Santa Monica, overlooking the famous Pier, and just a few blocks from our apartment.

"I should have gone right to the finish line and skipped the rest of the race," I say sarcastically. "It would have saved time."

"Let's get your bag checked in," says the ever-helpful David, still ignoring my snide remarks.

David's got more than a petulant passenger on his mind this morning. As an established running coach in the L.A. area—he oversees a group called USA Marathon Training—he has 36 other runners competing today. He has a booth set up just past mile

21—a few feet away from the Hirshberg booth, which is where I'm supposed to be stopping, taking photos and meeting with some of the real heroes of the race, pancreatic cancer survivors, many of whom have become my friends.

At the moment, however, I'm still not in a friendly mood. It's dark and cold, which just adds to my discomfort. Fortunately, I've been invited to hang out pre-race in Hirshberg's box inside Dodger Stadium -- like many of the race's big charities, they get to use a corporate suite so that their fund-raising runners have a warm, comfortable place to hang out before the race. David and I make plans to rendezvous at the start—about 90 minutes from now—and I make my way into the Stadium, down the corridor, past the giant pictures of Brooklyn and Los Angeles Dodger base-ball stars of the past and present—Hello, Jackie Robinson, hello, Clayton Kershaw!—and into the Hirshberg suite, marked by a sign.

"Julie!" says the perky staffer at the door when she sees me. "What is this...103?"

I've met her before, she's really nice, but at this hour and in my cross state of mind, I can't remember her name.

"Actually, 104," I say with a crooked grin. "But who's counting?"

Despite my mood, I'm polite. These are good folks, most

of them volunteers, and the cause, of course, really matters to me.

As I enter the suite, I see a gaggle of people crowded around the spread of food set up on a table near the door. Some of them are in race garb like me. I'm not ready to engage in small talk, so I grab a bagel and coffee and retreat outside the suite. Sitting in the hushed stadium, I gaze out at 56,000 empty seats. I then close my eyes, and repeat my mantra. I learned this from a good friend of mine, a TM teacher, who thought it would help me during the last stressful weeks of my 52-for-52 effort. It did. And I've practiced it daily ever since.

I push back the intruding thoughts—the doubts, the grumpiness, the "why-am-I-doing this?"

Hippy-dippy as it may sound, when I meditate, the mantra—an essentially meaningless word repeated over and over—gets rid of all the crap and all I'm left with is love. Sitting there, eyes closed, I realize that I love what I'm doing. I love the marathons, loved my dad, I love meeting and encouraging people, I love David and I love the fact that what we're doing is helping to fight, and maybe someday cure, a horrible disease. It's the only way I can do this, the only way I can be successful... and in my opinion, the only way anyone can ultimately be successful.

You have to be coming from love.

Feeling a little brighter, I walk back into the Hirshberg suite. The perky volunteer rushes over, with a young couple in tow. They're wearing light, breathable fabrics, flashy, multicolored shoes, and GPS watches on their wrists that can probably play videos. He's nibbling on a Clif Bar and she's sipping from a torpedo-sized water bottle.

Yup, they're runners.

"Julie," she says, "Todd and Shari are big fans of yours."

"Hi, guys!" I said, perking up. "Great to meet you."

"We love what you're doing," says Shari, smiling, as Todd nods earnestly. "This is our first marathon. I can't believe that you've done over a hundred."

"Neither can I!" I said, rolling my eyes theatrically. "But hey, your first one... that's exciting! Don't go out too fast!"

That's what we're always told—and of course, it's exactly the advice I ignored in my first few marathons. The adrenaline, the anticipation just seems to sweep you up. But you pay for it later. That's why David makes sure that I'm starting in the back today; so that I don't get carried away by either enthusiasm or, I guess, excessive crabbiness.

As I leave the suite, and head out to rendezvous with him, the sun is just beginning to rise. A few people in the crowd recognize me.

"Yo, Marathon Goddess!" says a short, muscular man with a crew cut. He offers me an upturned hand. We exchange high-fives. "I saw you on TV!"

"Julie, you are so inspirational," says a woman who approaches me with two of her friends, all wearing identical pink shirts. "I gave money after I heard you speak at the expo last year."

It's thrilling to hear this and, just like the ripening of the Southern California morning, I feel my mood lifting. Cranky Julie Weiss who needed more sleep is transforming into her alter ego. "Hey, everybody, c'mon," I yell out as we take our place in the starting corral, raising my arms wide. "It's going to be a great day!"

"Remind me of that at mile 23, Julie," says one wag.

No doubt running a marathon is hard. I think I sometimes make it look like too much fun. But if you're not enjoying yourself at least a little, I figure, why do it? In *Spirit of the Marathon*, one of the scenes that people tease me about the most occurred late in the film, in the final miles of the Rome Marathon. A little old Italian runner dressed in orange finally had enough of my constant chattering, exhorting, and cheering.

"Be quiet," he said to me in Italian—or at least that's how

the subtitles read. I think the producers were being kind in the translation. What I think he really said was "Shut the hell up, already, you annoying American!"

He looked up at me, continuing to scold me in Italian. "Don't talk! It will make you tired."

I didn't know exactly what he was saying, but I knew that I was being reprimanded. I didn't really shut up and it didn't matter. After we crossed the finish line, he hugged and kissed me.

I'm not alone in my lighthearted approach to a serious exercise in cardiovascular fitness. In the field at today's L.A. Marathon are runners dressed as cars and hot dogs; a guy wearing lederhosen; Elvis impersonators and Aztec Sun Gods—not to mention one self-proclaimed Marathon Goddess, whose sunny side is finally up.

A cheer in the distance, and suddenly the pack is moving, on our way out of Dodger Stadium. The race is starting! "Woohoo!" I yell, David at my side with a grin on his face. He'll peel off in a few minutes, and drive over to mile 21 to cheer his runners on. At my pace today, and with the minimal training I've mustered over the preceding weeks, I don't expect to get there for a few hours.

That's okay, because I'm feeling great now.

"You rock!" yells a bearded guy with a baseball cap.

"Thanks, have a great race!" I call back.

Now the speakers are pumping out the L.A. Marathon's signature song, Randy Newman's "I Love L.A."

We transition from walking to very slow jogging, the pack uncoiling gradually like a Slinky through the stadium's cavernous parking lot. I sing along with the call-and-response chorus of the 1983 tune that is now played at just about every major Los Angeles sporting event.

"Victory Boulevard...We love it!"

"Santa Monica Boulevard...We love it!"

I add my own line, raising my hands over my head, as I belt it out.

"L.A. Marathon...We love it!"

The strides get longer, the pack begins to open up and my spirits are soaring higher than the peaks of the San Gabriel Mountains. My heart is full, and somewhere, I like to believe, Maurice Weiss the drumming prodigy is keeping time to the rhythms of his daughter's pace. Slowly, but exuberantly, I'm on my way to another finish line.

I know it won't be my last.

Chapter 1
A Family of Performers

Long before this running obsession started--before the yearlong quest to run 52 marathons in 52 weeks, a different race each weekend, the aches and the heartaches, finish lines blurring together, the grind of my day job in between—I knew the joy of running but never recognized it. That joy was buried in my childhood so deep that I would never think that running would be how I would stitch the wound in my relationship with my father or heal my grief when he died. But it was always there, waiting to be rediscovered.

I remember it now: being a kid in the Southern California

hills, running through fields, my long legs flying over grass and my stringy blonde hair blowing behind me. That's when I started running.

My mom still owns my childhood home in Cheviot Hills on the west side of Los Angeles. It's nothing fancy, a Spanish-style, three-bedroom where my sister and I grew up amidst the ongoing soundtrack of my father's bands. Dad converted the garage into a soundproof recording studio and named it Leaky Roof Studios.

My mom, Bonnie, a prodigy on the piano at the age of four, channeled her rhythm and ear into modern dance. She's a woman whose every movement is a dance, a beautiful, lithe body with a soul of light.

Inside our living room, I'd listen to her play the concert piano from my spot on the Aztec-style carpet. Her hands flew across the keyboard and her long brown ponytail draped down her back. I was mesmerized by her music and her dancing. She flowed through her movements in long dresses, and you could feel her sweetness, her affection radiating through her limbs. Our mother was our protector—a woman who cradled you in her arms when you needed it the most.

My sister took up singing and I fell in love with the theater. I loved the energy of being on stage. We were free spirits living what looked from the outside like a perfectly normal SoCal life. And out in the Leaky Roof Studio garage, my father practiced with his brothers and his Dixie land band. It was hot jazz, "Muskrat Ramble," "Tin Roof Blues." Loud horns, string bass, and the booming voices of men singing kept me up at night. They always had a party to go to, an event to play. My father, who stood tall over everyone at 6' 3" could take up any room with his presence. Like his father, he was a drummer and he was also a master of the trumpet and piano.

My grandfather, Sammy, wasn't just any drummer. He was a jazz legend in the 1930's and '40's, playing with the likes of Louis Armstrong, Artie Shaw, Benny Goodman, and Tommy Dorsey. He grew up in the Lower East Side of Manhattan and taught himself how to play the drums at 3, using chair rungs as drumsticks and piecing together a drum set out of whatever he could find. He spent his teenage years playing weddings and events but came into prominence in the New York City jazz and swing scene of the early 1930's. Around that time, he met my grandmother and the pair fell madly in love. He was playing drums for the Benny Goodman Orchestra when they went on the road in 1934, but my grandfather decided to stay home and start a family. My father, his eldest, and the rest of my aunts and uncles grew up in a house with all-night jazz sessions and celebrity musicians coming and going. Each one of the kids took up several different instruments and would play right alongside my grandfather and the other greats of the time.

Sammy Weiss continued performing on the east coast until 1945, but that year my father got terribly sick. It was asthma and doctors said my father was ill-suited for the air in the city and might not survive another winter. So my grandparents packed up their five children and moved across the country to L.A. Luckily, the Jack Benny Show was also moving to the west coast, and my grandfather was the drummer. Like others in Benny's circle, he became a well-known comedic sidekick, beloved by the nation. He streamed through people's black and white televisions. There wasn't much else to watch on T.V. back then, so the wholesome broadcast was the thing everyone knew. Excitement would swell, in every living room across the country, as the jingle played. A man with a deep baritone voice announced, with a crescendo, the Jack Benny Show. And there was Sammy, the big guy, with the big voice, gently tapping his drums, and often playing straight man to Benny's humor.

The Benny show wasn't my grandfather's only gig. Sammy hosted a radio show called "Jammin' With Sammy," played with Dean Martin at the Coconut Grove, and was in "The Joker Is

Wild" with Frank Sinatra. He was an icon, both on the screen and in his family.

But the joyful musician and entertainer was not the man my dad saw at home. There, Sammy was miserable, filled with a brewing rage. Love and empathy were foreign concepts between father and son in that day and age, but the level of coldness my father felt from his dad went even deeper. Perhaps Sammy blamed the move out west on my father—and not just his medical condition. Despite his high-profile career, money was a persistent issue for Sammy. And so, every financial downturn was Maurice's fault. It was a pressing and ever-present guilt. On top of that guilt, my grandfather pressured my dad to succeed. He didn't want to see his oldest son follow in his musical path and face the same financial insecurity he was always battling.

I am not sure how harsh my grandfather was to my dad because he was never clear about it. Were there beatings? He vaguely mentioned how bad things got, but no one else in the family could confirm the hostility between Maurice and Sammy.

My grandfather is a shadow in my memory. I recall him bringing jelly donuts to our home every Sunday, announcing himself with his loud, jovial voice, the sun glinting off the top of his bald head, but that's really all. Still, his legacy lived on in our home through the name he made for himself in music and the whispers of his hot temper and the hell he gave my father as a kid. And while everything might have seemed like a golden dream in my own music-filled life, whatever abuse my father endured crept into the edges of our home.

My parents fought. A lot. Mostly about money and about how my father spoke to my sister and me. My instinct became to keep the peace and try to make everyone happy, especially my father. I wanted so badly for him to love us and accept us. And he did, he just didn't know how to express it. Instead of hugs, he took us on trips, letting me drive a boat down the Seine at age nine, renting a giant R.V. to go to the Grand Canyon. His trumpet came everywhere with us and he played for other campers or curious foreigners and made new friends. That was him in his element: gregarious, generous with his music, and amicable when he was on stage.

I remember long road trips in our car with our camping gear packed in the trunk. There was one in particular that I cannot forget on a dark road returning from whatever woodsy adventure we had just endured. It was tense in the car as my father grew agitated with me for something I cannot even remember now. I must've been five. He'd stopped the car on the side of the camp road and we idled there--me in the backseat with my older sister's eyes wide on me, my mother looking straight ahead into the distance. My father, all 230 pounds of him, seemed to be inching from the driver's seat to the back where I sat, and he was yelling.

"Julie!" The boom of his voice echoed around our car and out into the woods. He demanded I get out.

"Out?" I whispered.

"Maurice," my mother said, protesting in her calm way, laying a hand on his shoulder, urging him to turn around and keep driving.

"Get out of the car now," he said.

My sister began to cry. I looked out the window at the great trees towering over us. His hand reached back to the door handle and opened the door. Was he really going to just leave me here? My mother was yelling now, telling him to calm himself now. But he was still glaring at me with his eyes like black slits. Fear propelled me out of the car and onto the side of the road. I stumbled out, unstable on my feet.

"What are you doing?" I could hear my mother say as she got out of the car with me. I heard the door slam shut and then the car shifting into drive. He drove away.

My mother, who was a teacher before she had children,

stayed home with us in the light-filled house. She was the kind one, our defender.

We weren't stranded long; when the car returned my body was still frozen in the same shocked position where he left me. My father stared straight ahead with his hands on the steering wheel. My mother hugged me tight.

"Oh, Julie," she said in a cracked, hoarse voice.

She hurried me back into the car and we drove in silence home to our normal home to live what seemed like our very normal life.

But I felt these things my father did deeply and I tried my best to be the perfect child. I looked up to him for love and affection that never came. I knew he always wanted a son and I could not fill that void. He left me feeling incomplete, like there was a hole in my heart, a piece of me I could not fix.

I spent hours outside in my yard. I'd run into the kitchen, out of the screen door, with the hinges squeaking and the clank of the handle behind me. I could hear my mom's humming from the kitchen window. Beautiful sweet songs from the Sound of Music that acted in stark contrast to my father's banging drums and blaring trumpet. Outside, bushes along the perimeter of our fence created little places to hide. I tucked myself under the leaves and branches, away from the world, waiting for my mother to find me.

She'd lead my sister and I on quiet adventures, out through the fields where I first learned to run. She remembers now that I never followed a straight line. My legs would burn as I ran in a zig-zag with her following behind me.

I liked to stop, touch the ferns, or get lost in the tall grasses. It is this aimlessness that defines me. For three decades, I wandered through life with that hole in my heart searching for affection, and it led me astray for a good, long time.

My father was tough, but he created a perfect nest for my sister and me. While his passion was music, his trade was finance. He worked as a stockbroker. Before he left for work, I'd run up and say goodbye.

"Papa!" That's what my sister and I always called him.

In elementary school, I daydreamed. My father's wanderlust kept us on the move, taking trips to beautiful places, like the Grand Canyon, Slide Rock State Park in Arizona. We would also go cherry picking together. He even took us to Canada where he rented a big 35-foot motor home. When I was supposed to be learning, I'd stare out the class window and think of the big redwoods, the vast sand deserts he'd brought us to. In middle school, his judgement of my sister and I grew more intense. I'd feel his eyes on me when we took our trips. Those insecure years, where your body feels alien and every sideways stare hurt; that's when he really laid into us about our looks. He would point out the chubbiness of my legs, my disproportionate chest. I'd try to protect my sister from his words, but they cut us like daggers.

One night at dinner at our favorite Chinese restaurant I interrupted my mom and dad, probably pointing out at a pretty tree outside the window and my dad kicked me under the table and I started to cry.

"How dare you?" My mother said. She ushered us out of the restaurant. "Come on girls, we are leaving. Maurice, you can walk home."

She tried to explain that he wasn't used to dealing with girls, and she tried, but failed, to explain the transformation from girlhood to womanhood and all the physical and emotional changes that entailed.

His criticisms didn't make me love him less. Instead, I wanted nothing more than to please him. I felt like I could become the perfect, smart beautiful daughter he desired—I just wasn't sure how.

I tried makeup.

I tried doing well in school.

I tried singing songs I knew he would like.

He would come home from work, looking stressed from his job. By eighth grade I was up to his shoulders, I wouldn't meet him at the door and greet him. I hid until dinner. None of my tactics to gain his affection worked. And so, the older I got, the more I looked elsewhere for love.

Chapter 2
All the Wrong Places

I remember the cockroaches the most. And the brown tub and the sinking floor of the shower. Then there were the sombreros hanging on the wall that belonged to my boyfriend's father. Some mornings, I thought I'd woken up in Tijuana, but I was really in Westwood in an unkempt duplex living with five other adults and my newborn baby, Frankie. I'd wake to his gentle, hungry cries and the clatter of too many people living in too small a space. The smell of rice and beans on the stove, leftover from the night before, wafted through the house. I'd rise up, make my way to my baby, comfort him, feed him, get him dressed, and love him until it was time to get myself ready for my bookkeeping job. I was 18 years old and already living the world-weary, desperate life of an impov-erished 30-year old trying to keep her baby alive.

Back then, I never wondered how I'd ended up being a teen mom living between my mother's house and my boyfriend's house, juggling a baby and a job. I was happy that I had my boy-friend, Frank, to myself, but still I hungered for love.

I met Frank two years earlier when I was 15 and he was 17. Despite him being my ex-boyfriend's best friend, I knew he was drawn to me. My best friend in the world was with me, a girl I'd known since grade school. Lisa and I went everywhere together, and when she saw Frank look at me, she elbowed me hard in the ribs.

"Look at him," she giggled. I caught her eye and silently told her to stop. I wanted to look sophisticated, not like a school girl. She quit laughing and we approached. I could feel him staring at me.

He was leaning against the wall of Perry's Pizza in Santa Monica Beach, with a crowd gathered around him. His thick pony-tail and dark skin, the way he drew people to him—I wanted to be the center of his universe, so that me and him could stand together while everyone else orbited around us.

"Who is that?" He said when he saw me, and he said it loud

enough for me to hear. I was still new to wearing a more rebellious skin. This was only my second time sneaking out my bedroom window to meet friends. Lisa was new to this life too, and nervous. I drifted away from her tension and towards this boy who seemed so calm and self-assured.

The moon floated above the ocean, lighting the sky. It was an instant connection. His desire drew me in. It was curiosity for me—like a girl lost in the woods finding a black cave and thinking it might offer safety and a respite from the cold, lonely forest. He smelled like pot, but there was something else too—sandalwood, a deep and heavy aroma that clung to his hair. I liked his hair and his broad shoulders. The attraction was there.

He asked me to hang out with him the very next day, and I agreed. I told him to pick me up on the corner near where I lived. I would be waiting there. I wouldn't let him come to my house for fear my parents would see and lock me inside. Even without knowing him well, I could tell he represented danger—a world my parents had tried to shelter me from. I saw this as a means to escape from their world. It could not have been conscious at that point—I was young and naïve. But the thought of getting out of the house and into a loud car with a boy whose favorite activity was smoking weed at the beach seemed to be exactly what I needed. Get out,

out, out, my hormone-fueled brain urged me on.

In my small bedroom, I pulled on a jean skirt and a crop top. I flipped my head upside down and sprayed my hair with a toxic cloud of Sun-In. I found a pair of feather earrings and pair of slip-on vans, and quietly made my way to the door. My mother hummed and wiped counters in the kitchen.

"Where are you going, sweetie?"

"Out."

"With Lisa?"

"Yup."

"You'll be back for dinner?"

"Uh-huh."

I wasn't thinking past 30 minutes. I didn't know if I would be back for dinner, or ever. I didn't care. I stomped to the corner, wondering if Frank would actually show up. But I saw that car in the distance, and I broke into a trot. Freedom.

"Hey mama," Frank said. He sat behind the steering wheel, low in his seat.

His brother Fernando and one of his friends were in the car. My girlfriend told me his older brother was in a gang, and I watched him closely as he drank something golden from a paper bag. He offered me a sip.

"Sure."

It tasted bitter, awful. But I pretended I loved it.

Frank spoke in Spanglish to his brother, then translated for me. They both spoke English well but this was their natural language. I was the foreigner in the car, needing special sentences made especially for me.

"We're going to the hills," Frank said in his raspy voice, drawing out a long "e" sound in hill and hissing the "s."

I wanted to sound cool, nonchalant. I didn't have many fears, but I figured we would just be hanging out on the beach, where he usually loitered.

"What are we doing there?"

"Target practice."

Fernando laughed. I didn't know what that meant.

"I'm gonna teach you how to shoot a gun, mama," he smiled, and his mustache curled. "Cool?"

"Cool," I said.

We drove out of Santa Monica, on the highway, towards the Hollywood sign. I wasn't going to be back for dinner. Up into the woods, we continued driving with the sun lowering slowly, that yellow California orb protecting me from total darkness.

Frank pulled off in a little alcove in the bushes. He threw

the gear into park and we all climbed out. I looked around and saw nothing: just trees and leaves and golden hills.

"Grab some cans," Frank told his brother as he went around to the trunk. Fernando bent at the waist and collected soda and beer cans from the foot of the passenger's seat. He started tossing them out at my feet. I saw the tattoos on his arms and couldn't stop staring. When he picked up his head, he winked at me and smiled.

Frank got two shotguns out of the trunk of his car. They were long, clumsy things. The brothers spoke to each other at a rapid pace. Frank's friend, Ben was quiet. He leaned up against the car door sipping a coke and smoking a Marlboro.

"Can I have one?" I asked. He reached into his pocket and pulled one out. Then he held his lighter up and I smiled. I felt powerful with a cigarette in my hand. I held it more than I smoked it. And when I did inhale, a tiny cough gathered in my throat. I swallowed hard to keep it down.

"This way," Frank said and started walking on a trampled path. They'd been here before. We got to a clearing where spray paint marked the trees and old cans with bullet holes littered the ground.

"Ah, the great outdoors," Frank said. He spread his arms out like wings and let out a belly laugh. Fernando rolled his eyes.

"Frankie is always joking," he said. "Always a jokester, doesn't have a serious bone in his body, huh, bro?"

"I gotta have fun for the two of us, *hermano*," he held the gun up and looked through the scope.

"Don't worry, *mamacita*, it's not loaded."

Ben started lining up cans on a tree trunk.

"Okay," Frank said as he started loading bullets in the gun. "Now you're gonna stay back and watch for a second."

I stayed way back. I stood there in the clearing with my white sneakers and skirt, studying these boys with guns. Shots fired. Two loud booms, one right after the other. Frank was a good shot, his brother, even better. They laughed, studied their beer cans, admiring each other's aim. Ben took Frank's gun and had his turn. He had a shaky hand and missed the can.

"You're too soft, bro," Fernando said. "You have to be strong, hold the gun like it's your bitch and focus. Try again."

He missed the target again.

"Man, you're just wasting bullets," Frank said. He grabbed the gun back, too fast. I flinched and hoped he didn't see. Ben returned to his duty of lining up the cans. Frank and his brother repeated the process, laughing and whooping as they went. Then, Frank turned to me.

"Your turn," he said. "Come here."

I approached.

"You ever hold a gun before?"

"No."

"No problema. Here's what you have to do." He turned me around with his one hand near my waist and the other still on the gun. "Ok, keep your feet there. Now take the gun."

My hands felt like foreign creatures holding onto warm metal of this thing. I looked at him with wide, scared eyed. "No, girl, you got this." He helped me position it against my shoulder and stayed close explaining how to look through to the target. "Get your cheek right there close to it," he said.

"That thing is going to kick back so hard on her, she'll be off her feet," Fernando said. I looked up. He was laughing. "Ignore him," Frank said. "Shithead. Listen, it will be strong and you'll feel a little force come back on you when you pull the trigger. Just stay square on your feet, brace yourself."

I didn't know what he meant. He lined me up again, his rough hands moving up and down my arms, stroking my forearms and shoulders. I felt relaxed and anxious at the same time.

"Okay, ready?"

"Mhmmm," I didn't even want to breathe. I didn't want to

lose the position I was in.

"Ok, I'm gonna back up now." His hands left his body. I remained focused on the can. I heard my breath circling through my ears.

"Okay, ready, aim," Frank yelled. "FIRE!"

I pulled the trigger.

The gun kicked back against my shoulder, hard. I braced myself, held my breath, stayed square on my feet. When the smoke cleared, I let out a high-pitched whine. I hadn't even heard the shot; it was a moment of pure stillness, an incredible lapse in time.

"Damn," Frank was already over near the cans. "She hit one."

"Shut up," Fernando said.

"Look right here, bro."

I held the gun cradled in my arms, not knowing where to point it.

"Shit, she's a natural," Fernando said.

"That's a fucking turn on." The brothers laughed and slapped each other on the back. They called their friend Ben names and said he shot worse than a girl. I stood there as Frank took the gun back from me. He gave me a long hug. I stood, still in shock, smelling the gun powder on all of us.

I honestly didn't even know I was holding a real gun, a gun that could kill someone. The whole time, I thought it must've been a BB gun. I was shocked when Frank assured me it was real. And I was sore as hell—that kickback is no joke.

As I got closer to Frank, I learned he had an entrepreneurial spirit. He started working as a young kid delivering newspapers. He channeled that work ethic into dealing pot during his teen years. His three brothers joined gangs, but Frank did not. He was more into the surfing scene, and I grew enamored with his laid-back California attitude and the cloud of smoke that followed us wherever we went.

Shooting the gun set off something wild in me. Frank's friends became my friends, and I stopped going to high school. I kept in touch with Lisa and soon she was with us chilling out in 7-11 parking lots, asking adults to buy us beer. We would go to the beach. I loved this life. Although a part of me wondered what I was missing out on. I quit my modeling and acting classes. I felt I failed at that too, and somehow, I felt my boobs were too small, so I accepted this as my new life, with a longing in my heart. When I met Frank, I stopped everything.

One day, one of Frank's friends said she wanted to go shopping.

"Let's go," I said.

We didn't have any money, but Clarissa said that didn't matter.

"So you just want to look?" I asked. She was a tiny girl with dark hair and ruby red lips. She gelled her curls back into a tight bun that sat on the top of her head. We were a mismatched pair: she was barely 5-foot, and I had grown, again, since middle school. I was 5' 9" and towered over her, my lanky limbs gliding along next to her quick, fast steps. We headed towards downtown.

"Yeah, I just wanna look, I guess," she said. Lisa had gone to school that day and I was somewhat relieved. I knew she would want to come but would make me seem like a prude.

Our first stop, Nordstrom's at the Westside Pavilion near my parent's house. It was the middle of the day, on a weekday, and as soon as we walked in, I felt eyes on us. We weren't supposed to be in that store. My eyes were bloodshot from being at the beach all morning. I couldn't tell if the weed had made me paranoid, or if people actually knew that we were skipping school.

"I think we should go," I told Clarissa.

"Stop it, come on," she said.

I followed her as she made a loop around the first floor of the store. We zoomed past the handbags and the shoes, ignored the men's department.

"What are you looking for?"

"Not sure yet," she said.

We made our way past the cosmetics counters. We stopped at the perfume and Clarissa had me hold out my wrists so she could try different smells. Across from the perfume counter, I saw a pair of hoop earrings.

"Oh, look," I said to Clarissa. We drifted over to the racks of hanging jewelry.

"Those would look good with your outfit," she said. "Frank would like them. Get 'em."

I looked at the price tag.

"I don't have $50. I don't have any money, really." In my pocket, I had a five-dollar bill I was saving for a Slurpee. I had no business shopping.

"You don't need money, just take 'em," Clarissa said. I looked at her with my eyes wide. "Quit stalling. We've already been here too long. Just. Take. Them."

I glanced around. I felt dizzy. The fumes from the different scents Clarissa sprayed went straight to my head. At the Clinique counter, I saw a middle-aged woman watching us. Her hair was short and blonde, her glasses a ruby red. She was standing there, just staring.

"I can't."

"Oh my God, Julie, don't be a baby."

I took them. I tried my best to stuff them in my jeans pocket, but my pockets were small, and my jeans were tight.

"Let's go," Clarissa said.

I tried to explain that I hadn't yet secured the earrings, but it was too late. She was already taking her fast, pitter-patter steps to the front door. I lagged a few steps behind, the hoops burning indents in my palms.

"Miss?" A voice hissed from behind me. It was a man's voice and I heard the click-clanking of heels on the tile. I didn't turn around. Clarissa broke into a sprint. My breath got tight and just as I opened up my stride, I felt a hand on my shoulder. I was mere steps to the door. Clarissa was already outside, not looking back.

"Should I get the other one?" It was a security guard who had me by the shoulder.

"No," a woman's voice said. I shut my eyes. I knew it was the lady from the Clinique counter. "The tall one is the one who had them."

"Okay miss, where are the earrings?"

I opened my fist. Then I opened my eyes. I hoped maybe they would just let me go. I said I was sorry. That I really meant to pay…

"We've already called the police, miss."

They detained me in the back office of the store. The cops came and I sobbed uncontrollably. I was sorry, I didn't want to steal, but I was sorrier I got caught. Now, they would surely call my parents, who would find out that I wasn't in school and that I tried to steal earrings.

My mom picked me up. She didn't speak to me. I didn't try to explain, and she stared straight ahead at the road as we drove back to our home. I ran into my room and threw myself on the bed.

"Don't fall asleep, Julie," she called. "We're going to deal with this when your father gets home."

There was nothing I could say after that moment that would make my parents trust me again, so I figured, why try? What was the point of getting back in their good graces at this point, when the alternative was so much fun?

I kept sneaking out, stopped going to school. I didn't even try to hide it anymore. And I gained credibility within our group, too. Clarissa went back and told everyone that I got caught and almost arrested and I didn't snitch on her.

"Good girl," said Frank. "I'll get you those earrings if you really want them."

I didn't want them. I never wanted to go in a Nordstrom's again. But I liked the praise. I felt like I belonged. Being a perfect child had not worked out for me. I didn't gain the affection from my father I so badly wanted, so I replaced my obedience with defiance. Now I could fit into a new life with a new man. I would do anything for Frank. I wore my wild side like a badge of honor because I was Frank's girl and all I wanted was someone to love me.

The police seemed to like Frank, too. He and his family and friends were easy targets for the cops. We spent a lot of time out on Frank's street, just messing around. One winter night, a group of us were outside, sitting on the sidewalk, taking a break from watching a football game inside Frank's dad's home. The police drove by us then looped back around. I was thrilled. Frank was annoyed.

"They're always up and down this block," he said, angrily.

"Calm down," his father, Papa Henry said. He was always the voice of reason and he welcomed everyone into his life with love, even the cops. He was a good, hardworking man, a janitor at UCLA who raised all five of his children on his own. His wife left him when Frank was just five weeks old. The aunts and uncles of the family wanted to split the kids up, take in one or two, but

Papa Henry insisted his family stay together. It was a full house, with friends of his children always in and out. And the police were always checking in.

"Why are they here, we ain't doing anything," Frank said.

When the cars stopped this time, they got out of the car and demanded we line up by the curb.

"We're not doing a thing," Frank said. He was telling the truth. They shined the spotlight on us and looked us up and down, searching some of the boys. Of course, at this moment, my father drove down the street and slowed to a crawl. He was most likely checking up on me. I probably mentioned around where Frank lived. He just randomly drove by. It was weird, but not out of character. This is how he met Frank's family: Lined up and spread-eagled against a fence in the barrios.

And then, days later, he officially met Frank. We were riding home from the beach in an old Pinto, passing a joint back and forth. My father was waiting for me outside our family home with his hands in his pockets, ready for my arrival. Maybe I was too high to care, or maybe I just truly didn't give a damn, but I opened that Pinto door and emerged in my bikini with the joint still blazing and a cloud of smoke following me.

"Get the fuck out of here," my dad said to Frank. Frank just looked at me, looked at him, nodded and hit the accelerator. My father sent me to my room and I laughed. "My room? Please, I'm not 10 years old."

I waited until my parents went to bed and I snuck out my window, stole my father's 1969 Pontiac convertible Firebird and drove back to Frank.

Still, I wasn't happy. Even with Frank in my near-constant sight, I was petrified he would cheat on me. Everyone loved him, especially his ex-girlfriend who was adorable, and blonde, and had really big boobs. The thought of losing Frank made my stomach ache and pulse in pain. I was 16 and the only thing I could think of was Frank and making him mine forever.

Lisa was the only person I could talk to about this. She always said I was being crazy.

"Chill out, Julie," she said when we were together and Frank wasn't with us. "Every girl would die to look like you, and Frank knows he has the best."

Lisa was shorter and rounder than me but just as beautiful. She didn't seem to need the constant reassurance I did. I let her stroke my hair and tell me everything would be okay.

Other girls in the neighborhood were having babies at a rapid pace. Fifteen-year-olds had toddlers, girls my age were on their second child. I started to feel old to be a mom—at 16! Many of them asked me when I planned to have a baby. This sparked an idea in me. Secretly, I stopped taking my birth control pills.

When I told Frank I was pregnant, he didn't look surprised.

"Okay, we'll have a baby," he said. He seemed happy, and perhaps he thought not much would change. I know that's how I felt.

What I know now is that the unconditional, undying love and family I was looking for from Frank was an attempt to fill the void that my father left. I chose a guy with charisma, whose personality could fill a room—just like my dad. Of course, he was the opposite in a lot of ways, too, but now I can see clearly the reason for my dependence on Frank and why I was so desperate to trap him. I never thought through what forever meant and I was unprepared for a baby.

Dad knew it. "You need to give the baby up for adoption," he said. It was his first reaction to the news. "You are 17 and a high school dropout. And now you're pregnant. How are you going to support this baby?"

Meanwhile, Papa Henry took me in. He bought me all the foods I wanted when I was pregnant. He was a jolly, warm, man. I sat with him in the den of their home every night and we watched

TV together, him with a Budweiser and me with whatever sweet food I could get my hands on. He taught me how to make home-made enchiladas and tamales. I was so happy for his love and acceptance.

But my dad was rational—and right. I had no plan at all as to how I would raise a child. But I wasn't going to give the baby up no matter how much my family panicked. Despite his initial criticisms, my dad wanted to help. He started thinking practically about what I could do, how I could handle the new responsibility I had added to my young life. He told me to start looking into book-keeping careers. It wouldn't be glamorous, but it would pay for diapers, so I listened. He also advised me to take some classes at Santa Monica Community College, and I did. I actually did really well in them.

When Frankie was born, my father softened. This was the son he'd always wanted, and Frankie became the center of my dad's universe. He looked just like my Dad. He was blonde, with piercing blue eyes. Even Frank thought this was the mailman's kid. But this little being brought everyone together, made peace between Frank and my dad and all the family members I was sure would abandon me.

I got a 9 to 5 job as an office assistant and continued taking accounting courses at the college. Frank was trying to launch his own plumbing business (and was likely still dealing on the side). Lisa's dad owned a baby gym, and I took Frankie there all the time. She was a ray of light, tickling Frankie and loving him like an aunt. She and I worked out together, doing an amazing amount of aerobics; I was on a mission to lose the baby weight and she wanted to get in shape. Frank and I had a little money, our health, our friends, our baby, and a place to live, thanks to Papa Henry.

Despite the mess inside Frank's home, his family was kind and generous. Papa Henry became a stand-in for my own dad. We ate together, laughed together, and I basked in the warmth this large family provided. For a little while, everything felt good, almost normal. But I was like a flower, just blowing in whatever direction the wind took me, growing only where the sunlight shined. I knew in my heart that it could all fall apart in a moment, I just wasn't sure when this little life I'd created would start to unravel.

Chapter 3
Into the Flames

I wanted to make it work.

Frank was in love without knowing how love was supposed to work. I kind of loved Frank, but I didn't know what love was, and I liked the idea of having a man. Trust didn't exist between us. On nights out, at concerts or restaurants, Frank would start fights with men who dared look at me. In a strange way, I felt honored. I thought he loved me enough to protect me. But most nights, I wasn't out with Frank. I was 21 years old, at home with Frankie, who was three years old already, worrying about who he was talking to—what girl was on the bar stool next to him. I was certain he was cheating on me and I wanted to catch him red-handed. We wanted all of each other, at any cost.

On an ordinary night, I fed Frankie. Then I would wait for

Frank to get home, we would eat, and he would head back to the bar. I read my baby a bedtime story and scratched his head until he fell asleep then tried my best to make myself busy around the house. I finished the dishes, wiped down the counters, ran through a list of what I had to do at work the next morning, washed my face, then checked the clock. It was 9 p.m. Where was Frank? His schedule was never predictable, but now I was home with our baby and I knew what he was likely doing--hanging out, drinking, being the life of the party. I tried to relax. I talked myself down. I knew who he was and he loved me, right? He wouldn't betray me like that.

Another hour, more waiting. I couldn't take it. It was another late night and I didn't want to go to bed alone again. I wandered into the Frankie's darkened room.

"Frankie," I whispered, lifting him up and drawing him close to my chest. "Come on, just wake up for a little bit. We're just going to take a ride."

"Where are we going?" He asked. He rubbed his eyes. He was so small and yet he seemed to understand I needed him at that moment.

"We just have to pick up your Dad," I said, trying to sound calm, normal.

I loaded him into his car seat and pulled away from our little home, a house that Frank's aunt had bought for us. What was I doing? Driving the streets at 10:30 p.m., visiting Frank's regular spots. Bars, haunts, friend's homes, I drove to all the places I thought he might be, trying to catch a glimpse of his car. I knew it was crazy, that this behavior was totally nuts. I knew letting him control me in this way was unhealthy for me and my child. By 11 p.m., I was tired. I looked in the rearview at Frankie sleeping in the back seat and felt sick. I couldn't find Frank. I wasn't going to catch him in some sinister act. Even though I felt like he was cheating on me with every fiber in my being, I didn't have proof and I didn't even know what I would do if I did. We returned home. Frank still wasn't home, but I had worn myself out. It wasn't the last time I would go out on a late-night expedition to find him.

I never caught him in the act, but finally what I thought was happening was confirmed. Friends told me. Frank had cheated. With my best friend. Lisa.

Once I finally knew it to be a fact, I couldn't handle the gut-wrenching pain. I packed up Frankie.

"Where the hell are you going with my son?"

"What do you care?"

"You can't just take him and leave," he shouted.

"You cheated on me! With my best friend. She was the only person in the world I trusted. You asshole!"

Papa Henry watched us fight and held Frank back as I took off out the door and back to my parents.

I swore it would be the last time, that I would never return. There had been other breakups, but I promised him this time I meant it. He was sorry, he said. At first, I shrugged off his apologies. But I couldn't stay away. He was the father of my child. It was stupid, but I went back to him. I always went back.

We gave birth to our second child, Samantha, in 1993. We got hitched in 1995. Even at 25, I was still too young to know how marriage was supposed to work. He was 27 and we tried our best, but we'd spent our early twenties as babies raising a baby and we never grew up ourselves. Then, about a year into our marriage, Frank got arrested. Again. He was always getting arrested for DUIs, dealing weed, expired registration and warrants. You name it. His 1967 blue Chevy Malibu with no muffler, his long hair flying out the window and drinking beers while driving just made him an easier target. While on probation for one thing or another, he got caught with weed and was sentenced to one year in prison. Other stints in jail had been shorter and I was able to survive, and in fact thrive without Frank in the house. Each time he got sent away, my life flourished. The kids and I were a cohesive unit and I excelled at my job and in my classes without the distraction of a husband I didn't trust. I was sad he would be gone for such a long time, sad for the children who would have to visit their father in prison, and sad for Frank who was young and stupid, but not a criminal. Still, I knew I had to keep going to provide for our family.

My parents helped, of course. They were my rock during unsteady times and kept their doors and hearts open no matter what. I continued working, trying to make my dad proud by spending long hours perfecting my work and advancing quickly. Nothing was perfect in my life. How could it be with a husband in jail? But it was manageable.

Frank's friends were still my friends and we hung out when I wasn't working and the kids were with my parents. There was a house party one night with our old group and I swung by. I stood in the driveway with some old friends, drinking a cold beer with the cool California breeze blowing through my hair. I noticed him then, a man in the garage, sitting on a stool, watching me.

"Who is that?" I asked.

I walked into the garage and wandered back towards him. He watched my every move. I liked his eyes on me. I liked that raw desire he didn't bother hiding. I'd later learn that his name was Johnny and he was of Italian descent. When he stood up, he was quite short, 5"5'. But that didn't bother me. I wanted to get to know him and we started a friendship even though I knew his intentions by simply reading his gaze.

When Frank was released, I tried so hard to get us back on track. I ignored the insecurities that plagued our relationship--the fact that he cheated on me, the terrible possessiveness that led him to assault other men. Instead, I bought new carpets for the house. I bought some furniture. I thought of it as a new beginning, but I was just filling a deep void with material things.

Meanwhile, Johnny lurked in the background. I was drawn to him like a magnet. He was kind of sexy, with his dark energy and beautiful face, but the fact that he was so attracted to me made me excited. Frank had cheated, I reasoned, so I slowly started to succumb to Johnny's advances. I wanted out of my marriage--out of the house where I felt broken--and I wanted a new life with this new man.

Johnny was different than Frank. Johnny was passionate and fun-loving. "Julie, my *bella donna*," he'd say whenever he saw me. His parents had immigrated from Italy, but Johnny had been born here. Still, he could speak the language in a delicious voice that made me tingle.

He had baggage, too--an ex-girlfriend with whom he had a daughter and deep moods that I didn't fully understand. He lured me in with his charisma and charm and I fell hard.

Our affair took off quickly after Frank and I decided to separate. I spent long hours with Johnny, hungry for his desire. Johnny had a place a few miles away in the San Fernando Valley, but in those miles my life was completely different. While the kids stayed safe with my parents, I went out at all hours partying and trying to fan the flames of this new romance.

On dark corners, under the dull haze of streetlights, I'd huddle into phone booths to make calls for drugs.

"I think we need a pick-me-up," he said. "I'm getting bored and tired. Let's go dancing, let's go anywhere but home."

Johnny had a taste for cocaine, and sometimes crack. I tried it. He didn't really force me. I learned how to cook the cocaine so that it would turn into rock, and we smoked it together. I was a love addict, and so whatever I could do to be with him, I did. I tried it and liked it. For a little while those highs helped me feel unstoppable. I ignored the heartache of a failed marriage and the acute sense that I was ruining my life.

One late night, in a dazed state, we strolled his neighborhood together, hand in hand. Johnny was in a particularly good mood and feeling spontaneous.

"Wanna get a tattoo?"

"Sure," I said. Why not?

We followed the neon lights to a dark, cold shop.

"We'll get each other's names," he said.

I laughed. But he was serious. It happened quickly. He was already in the chair, his shirt off, the font chosen, the sketch applied to his bare chest.

"I'm getting my tongue pierced," I called over my shoulder as I followed a young dude with ink covering every inch of his body into a booth across the way. I decided to put his name on the back of my neck in a classic cursive. It felt like hot razor blades poking holes in my spine. What the fuck am I doing? I thought. Another thought ran through my mind: You're getting branded. But I tuned out and buried my head deeper into the plastic table. I accepted the pain, this was who I was now.

I rode the highs, but some mornings, Johnny would be different, and everything would come crashing down. His rage seemed endless.

After putting the kids to bed late one night at my Mom's house, I left, dying to see Johnny. I went to the liquor store and made a call to get some cocaine then drove straight to his home.

I knocked on his door.

When he opened it and saw me, he slammed it in my face.

I didn't understand. What had I done? Was he mad at me?

I knocked again.

"Get the fuck out of here you ugly bitch!" His voice, which was once so smooth and inviting, sounded sinister.

I should've been mad, but I was embarrassed. And rejected. I crumbled in front of the door and cried.

"I can hear you out there," he raged. "I will come out there and make you fucking leave."

I scurried onto my feet and ran from the door. I didn't want to be hit and I didn't want to make him more mad at me.

"Bitch!" he called after me. I had no idea what was going on with him. I couldn't figure out.

I drove away in the dark, but soon pulled over crying hysterically. I paged him over and over. He wrote back in pager code, "Go to HELL."

I vowed never to go back.

But I did go back. Over and over. He would love me, then spit me out and love me and spit me out. I kept going back and accepting his apologies because that was my drug of choice--the illusion of love.

I was alone with him on Christmas morning in 2000. When I woke up, a cold, gray sun shined in my face and I looked over at Johnny's side of the bed. He wasn't there. I stumbled out in my pajamas and headed out to see what he was doing. There was a smell--something chemical--gas. He was face down on the couch, unmoving.

"Johnny?" I said. Nothing. His lips looked blue and his face, usually tan, looked pale.

"Johnny!" I yelled. Nothing. The smell filled the room. My head started to spin. I walked to him.

"Johnny!" I yelled again, shaking him. "What are you doing?"

"Get off me," he said. "I want to die."

He was trying to kill himself, attempting to fill the house with gas from the stove, while I was still there, on Christmas morning. I turned off the gas and opened all the windows.

I tried hugging him. He wouldn't let me touch him. "Get the fuck off me," he said.

I called his sister to tell her what happened and let her know I had to get out of there. He wanted me to leave too. Dumbstruck, I drove to Santa Monica beach and stumbled to the place I first met Frank, lifeguard tower 26. I dropped to my knees, like Jimmy

Stewart in "It's A Wonderful Life."

"Please God," I pleaded. "Help me." But unlike the movie, no lovable angel named Clarence appeared. We just continued on with the dysfunctional grind of our lives.

I stayed with him, even after that. In my weakened, drugged-out state, it never occurred to me that I had the freedom to just leave.

Two months later, Frank called to tell me his father was going to die.

"It's cancer," Frank said over the phone. I was devastated. I remembered the kindness his dad always showed me, how much he loved my kids, the food he made for us all. I missed that kind of love.

Papa Henry had been living in Utah with his daughter at the time and Frank was organizing a trip so we could see him before he passed away. I got off the phone and told Johnny I needed to go with Frank on a trip to see his ailing father.

No. That was his answer. No.

I didn't understand. I wasn't asking permission. I asked him what he meant. He told me that he meant, no. I couldn't go. There was no way he would let me travel with my ex-husband to another state. I couldn't believe it.

"What do you mean I can't go?"

"I'm not letting you go on vacation with your ex-husband in Utah. Are you kidding me?"

"This isn't a vacation." I couldn't believe he said that.

"I know you're cheating on me, I just never thought it would be with that guy. I thought you left him for me."

"You're being crazy."

"Call me crazy one more time, you slut."

He grabbed my arm and pulled me towards him. He was crazy, and he was hurting me.

It was as though my eyes had finally opened. What was I doing in this relationship? Everything in my life was being controlled by this unstable man who didn't actually love me, let alone care about me. I left immediately. I took whatever I could out of that house—it wasn't much that I could grab, but I didn't care.

This would be the last time, I promised myself. I'd neglected my family long enough because Johnny said he needed me. And his cruelty was only getting worse.

I left, and this time for good: I never went back.

Frank, me and our kids went to Utah to say goodbye. When we got home after our visit, there was a call to say Papa Henry had passed. He had waited for us.

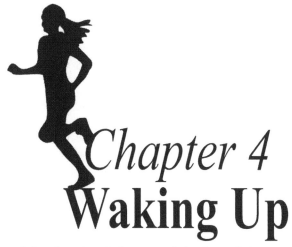

Chapter 4
Waking Up

After leaving Johnny and the late nights and drugs behind, things were supposed to get better. I was supposed to be better. I had made the decision to change my life and take care of my family. That's how the story is supposed to go, right?

I left Johnny in 2000. Over the next six years, I raised my kids, held down and excelled in my work—doing accounting for Johnny Rockets and then Wolfgang Puck's. I moved out of my parent's home and my kids and I settled into a nice little house just a few minutes away from them. It was a little shabby, but still had a homey feel to it. Hardwood floors, a bright kitchen, and the kids each had their own room. I took the strange little covered patio in the back as my room. It was enclosed, but kind of funky. Our home was sandwiched by million dollar mini-mansions and my son complained it was the ugliest house on the block. But it was a house and I made it a home. I even got us a puppy named Jessie.

I dated here and there, still getting sucked into terrible relationships, but I now had the foresight to get out quickly. Even though I'd grown up, there was still this longing. Deep down, I knew that I wasn't fulfilling that potential. Instead of trying to search for it, I started to feel more and more worthless. I went through the motions of everyday life with a darkness following me. *Why am I here,* I wondered. *I am fat, worthless, horrible. I have nothing to be proud of.*

When tax season rolled around in 2005, my spirits lifted slightly. In my line of work, tax season is like the Olympics. I loved the rush of getting the work done--numbers flying, forms complete. Being busy kept my mind from wandering. I wasn't asking if there was supposed to be more to life. No, I was hustling to get my work done living on the high of getting through the workload and having even more to do on my desk the next day. It fed my addictive nature. I was hooked on the work, the late nights spent at my desk, and the accomplishment of truly hard work.

In the few months of filing, I soared. Then after April 15, when it was over, emptiness took over. Something broke inside me. The dark thoughts returned, the introspective musings on a life that seemed to have gone very wrong. I'd show up to my job and sit at my desk, blankly. Soon, more thoughts invaded. Thoughts of suicide, of ending it all.

The last time I thought like this was back in the Johnny days. I couldn't believe this type of pain was returning. I only thought such hurt could be caused by a broken heart, by a sick man not returning my phone calls. Back then, in my mother's house, coming off of all the coke and crack, I had swallowed a handful of sleeping pills and hoped for pain to stop. It was a cry for help—and thankfully not enough to kill me. I slept for two days and woke up knowing that I wouldn't do that—I had kids and people who loved me. But now, the darkness was bearing down on me again and I still had those old, expired pills tucked away in my closet somewhere.

That morning when I took my dog Jessie for a walk, I saw this group of people on the beach. They were happy and there were thousands of them. They looked athletic and they were all shapes, sizes, colors, milling about and talking to one another. Then they formed little groups and one by one, they took off running. As each group took off, I felt this pang of hurt mixed with extreme joy. I was so happy for them. They were doing something so beautiful, together. But it was as though there was a wall built between me and them--like a barrier that I couldn't break through. I would never be able to be part of something that beautiful. I felt alone. Jessie had looked up at me and her eyes seemed to understand the hurt I felt, and I just cried. Remembering those runners, and Jessie, and thinking about my family and how I was nothing more than a shell of a person bothering them—failing them all in one way or another, I thought about the sleeping pills. It was a relief to think of them—to think about taking all of them.

I didn't have an exact plan. Not a day or time, but I couldn't stop thinking about ending my own life. In the morning one Saturday, my dad came over to my place. I wasn't expecting him to visit and the house was a mess. Piles of laundry sat next to the washer in the kitchen. The dishes in the sink were crusted with food and piled high. My light-beige cabinets and counters were a sickly gray. I sat at the table in the middle of the room and waited for him to come in.

"Julie!" My dad beamed. "Hello."

He didn't mention the mess. He looked past the stains on the linoleum floor and the remains of last night's dinner in the sink. It's not that I didn't want to clean, it's just that everything felt overwhelming. I looked up at him from where I sat and blinked away tears.

"What's wrong?" He asked. He was quiet and concerned.

"I'm just so…" I could hardly finish the sentence. What could I say? I feel hopeless and that life isn't worth living? That I have nothing? That this wave of blackness had taken hold of everything in my life and left me feeling exhausted, defeated, and numb?

"I'm just a little down," I said. I cried. He held my shoulder. "Didn't you..." I started. "Didn't you feel like this?"

My dad had bouts with depression, but it was not something he talked about. Mom had called it moodiness and he never mentioned it to anyone. He nodded, though. The light from the window poured in over us. I felt a little less alone.

"It's going to be okay, Julie," he said. "I love you."

It was the first time those words had ever come out of his mouth. I could feel his love in that moment and I trusted that he was right, maybe things would get better. I went to the doctor, who prescribed Effexor—Selective Serotonin Reuptake Inhibitor (SSRI) —for my depression. I was desperate and knew I needed help and so I took them without question. I started feeling a little better. Life seemed manageable. Together the kids and I continued going through our days. Even though I could get through work, the pills didn't help. I made all the unhealthiest choices. I worked some nights until 11 p.m. and dinner would often be fast food or ready-made meals. I gained major weight. I spent my 20's at about 115 lbs. But the antidepressants combined with eating terribly and being chained to my desk took its toll. I ballooned up to 165 pounds in two years, which of course, made me hate myself even more.

I know that many, many people need antidepressants to be their best selves, to keep living—but as the months went on, the meds made me strange. My job got harder. I felt like I was spinning my wheels in a place where the work was slightly above my head and where I was constantly being watched and micromanaged. I could've asked for help, but I didn't want anyone to know I was struggling. Anxiety took control of my body, and I started tearing at my skin. The picking is a nervous habit that I still do to this day, but back then, working late with stacks of paper sitting in front of me just waiting to get done, I would scratch the palms of my hands until they bled. I told my doctor about the darkness that hovered over me even with the pills, and his only solution seemed to be raising the dosage. My brain was flooded with serotonin at the highest milligram possible, and still, I felt lost.

My dad started planning a family trip to Hawaii in 2007.

By that time, I'd gotten sick of being heavy. I tried small changes. A co-worker and I made a pact to go on diets and I even tried dragging myself to the small park near my house a few times to walk. Sometimes, I lengthened my stride enough to call it a run--but just for a few seconds. Any movement left me feeling exhausted and defeated. When my dad told us to get ready for a vacation in Kauai, I made up my mind. This vacation would be my chance to turn it all around. I wanted to leave the skin I was in on the mainland and use the trip to reinvent my life.

As many family trips do, it started out rocky. Despite his nice gesture to bring us all together, he couldn't help but comment on my weight as we waited for our baggage in the airport.

"Wow, Julie, did you see how slim your sister looks?" he said, hinting not so subtly at my weight problem. "She looks fantastic. You should talk to her about what she eats."

I tried to ignore him, but his words cut. I knew I was heavy, I didn't need him to tell me that I had packed on even more pounds. He just couldn't help himself. My sister and my daughter argued about room selection, my mother threatened to fly home to avoid the drama, and my dad wandered around with his trumpet trying to stay out of it all.

Frankie, by then 17, had elected to remain home and at first,

I wished I'd stayed with him. I didn't try to fulfill my peacekeeping duties, I just let the arguments settle around me. The rooms were sorted out, my mom decided to stay, and I went to bed early, anxiously awaiting the sunrise.

That morning, I woke up and pulled on a white bikini. The only thing good about the weight was that my boobs looked bigger, which distracted me from the fact that my thighs looked like cottage cheese. I left the house and headed to the beach barefoot. I was going to run--to actually run. I was going to run like those people I saw on the strand. I also knew from beauty and fitness magazines that running would help me lose weight. The air in Kauai smells of Hibiscus blooms and salt air, and I filled my lungs to the brim. I was open to the universe, willing to accept whatever the moment wanted to throw at me. With the morning sun beaming down on the white sand, I made my way from the house to the shoreline. I couldn't describe the feeling or what had gotten into me. I wasn't prepared, and it didn't matter. I turned parallel to the ocean and its crashing waves and lifted one leg. And then the other.

What I remembered that morning was the freedom I felt running when I was little. The memories of my fingertips touching wild grass as I sprinted through fields, that was my hope. I thought if I could relive that, I could find happiness--not in my work, or my man, or a prescription--but in myself.

I heaved my leg up from the sand and made another step, then another. God, it hurt. I felt the sand cradling my bare feet and thought of my earliest memories, the apartment my parents rented when I was just born until I was three. It was in Malibu, right on the beach. There, my mother danced while watching the waves roll in and the tides ebb in and out, and everything was perfect. I'd always felt a strong connection to the shore, and now I was back in that perfect space where stress and the limitations of my body and mind did not exist. I kept trying to move forward, thinking to myself, I am really doing this, and I feel at home.

This wasn't the awkward running I tried to endure back in California. It wasn't trying to punish my body for racking up pounds. I was bounding over the obstacles that had led me to my current state of mind, feeling connected to the beach, to the earth, and accepting how hard this moment really felt. Physically, I felt like I might die. But something inside me had come alive.

I pushed myself through the run until I fell into the sand, my knees dropping into the earth. I remembered kneeling on the beach on Christmas Day when Johnny had tried to kill himself with me in the house and all the horrible things he'd ever said to me. There was a lifetime of trauma inside me.

I stood up from the sand, brushed off my legs, and tried to run a few more steps.

It wasn't far. Maybe I lasted a quarter mile, if that. But distance did not matter. I felt clear and plugged into life again. My lungs were exploding, and my legs wobbled. I felt like I might be dying, but I stumbled my way from the sand to the ocean and jumped in.

There is a place in Kauai where the mountain streams flow into the ocean, and the point where the two waters meet each other is supposed to be a place of great healing. I felt that moment as if I was the mountain stream. I had rolled down through the rocky terrain of my life all the way to this point, and as I mixed with the ocean, I felt refreshed, rejuvenated and I knew this was where my life was going to begin.

That night, without ceremony, I threw away the antidepressants.

I went out and ran every morning during our week-long vacation on Kauai. Each day, I went a little farther. Some of it was walking and some of it was running and sometimes I couldn't even stay on my feet. I'd get back to the beach house and find my dad. We'd stand on the deck and I would point in the distance to where I'd made it to that day. I would then drop down and hold a plank for about ten seconds.

"I'm going to get strong," I told him.

"Good job," he said. "But you've got a long way to go."

He always had to get a jab in somewhere. But I sensed the softness in his voice and understood something that I hadn't let myself feel before. He was genuinely proud of me. I was doing something for myself, and in his own way--by letting me point out the rock I wanted to run to by the end of the trip and by suffering through my unsteady planks with me--he let me know he was impressed.

I did make it to that rock. It felt like 10 miles, but I think it was actually about two. When I looked up to the patio on that last day, as I struggled for air on my run back to the rock, I saw two faces looking down on me. My mom and dad. They waved, then broke into a round of applause.

Returning home, I wasn't about to let myself lose the momentum I had created on the island. Everything felt new again. I didn't know what I was running from and I could not see where I was running to. I just knew that I could not stop.

Chapter 5
The Very
First Start Line

The day after I returned from vacation, I stepped out of my house, walked the five blocks to the beach, and stepped onto the sand. I breathed deep, trying to create the same sense of peace I got on the island. I can't say it wasn't hard to start. I had come home; back to a place where I felt like a failure for so long. Still, that energy I'd cultivated for myself in Hawaii charged through me. I told myself that I was allowed to feel healthy and to be happy. I took it all in again: the sand, the waves, the orange morning sun on my face. There was no turning back and no time to bring up all the bad times. I thought instead of my mom and dad and how just one week of changes had reignited their true pride in me, as though they saw that I was capable of more than just existing. My dad's face when I told him I'd made it to that rock looked like shock and pride. I'd set a goal, I did it, and he could hardly believe it. I wanted to make him--and the rest of my family--that proud of me all the time. And I wanted to feel better. In the near distance I spotted a lifeguard stand (or "tower" as we call them on the beaches of Southern California).

That was my first marker; my first finish line.

"Come on," I told my legs. "Let's go." I took off, wobbling in the soft sand, feeling my chest heave up and down. The lifeguard stand seemed so close, but it was taking forever to get there. I estimated that it was about a half-mile away from me and each step felt like an eternity. Gone was the adrenaline I had during the trip. I felt heavy and uncoordinated. I was kicking the insides of my calves, spraying sand up onto my legs, my arms, my face, and I wanted to stop. Of course, I didn't. When I reached the stand, I had sand covering every inch of my body. I couldn't catch my breath and I poured myself onto the structure waiting for my heart to calm down. Tomorrow, I thought, I'll make it to the next stand, and the next day, I'll go to the stand after that. The coastline stretched out in front of me like miles of possibilities. There would be no quitting.

Later that day, I swung down to the pool in my apartment complex. A neighbor, Kate, whom I was friendly with was sunbathing and I sat down to join her. I wanted to tell someone about my trip, and about running.

"You sound like Tony Robbins," Kate said, only half joking. I knew the Robbins craze well. When I was trying to pull myself out of the depression that was slowly swallowing me, I had read his books and tried my best to achieve personal growth. But she was right in one way. I was tired of settling.

"Yeah," I said. "I want my life to be extraordinary. I want to be extraordinary."

"Hell, yeah," she said. After a second, she shifted her body towards me. "Hey. Maybe we could run. Like together?"

"Let's do it!" We started planning the schedule. We both had dogs. My Jessie is a Golden Retriever, Collie, Chow mix. Kate had a Weimaraner. Both were about 3 years old with plenty of energy. We decided on taking them out for a beach run instead of their normal, morning walk. We decided to meet at the beach at 4:45 the next morning. I am an early bird, but not that early. This was a part of the new commitment. I loved it. Even if I didn't sleep well.

The dogs kept us going. I told her about my lifeguard station strategy and how if we made it to one stand, then we could certainly make it to all the others. She hadn't run a day in her life. And I only had about 10 days under my belt. But at our feet, the dogs waited patiently.

"Okay, Jessie," I said to my mutt. Jessie is not any mutt though, she is an amazing fluff ball. When we started, I knew she would love running. I just didn't realize how much she would embrace it as part of her, and our, lives. "Let's go."

I unhooked Jessie from her leash and Kate did the same. They sprinted, fast, away from us, rumbling in the sand and dipping their paws in the water. We didn't have time to over think it, we needed to follow them or else they'd end up in Catalina. Kate and I didn't chat. We just breathed hard and locked into making it to the lifeguard stands. We made it to two and back, gasping and pleading with the dogs to wait up.

"I thought you said this was amazing," she said at the end. She crouched on the sand and let her pup lick the sweat from her forehead. I didn't know what to tell her. I was pretty beat myself.

"Same time tomorrow?"

"I guess that's what we're doing," she said. "I hope it gets better."

Kate was out the next day, and the day after that. Meanwhile, I'd been telling everyone about running. I cornered anyone who would listen. My coworkers didn't know what to think of this new obsession. My family smiled as I told them about the different distances I was attacking. And one friend, Nina, a free spirit with a laid-back way about her, surprised me. She told me we should sign up for a triathlon.

I thought she was nuts. Here I was, struggling to run two miles at a time, and she wants me to commit to a race where I would not only run six miles, but bike and swim in the ocean, with waves, and with a crowd of crazed athletes in wet-suits. But it was only May, there was time. So, I figured, why the hell not?

The weight started peeling off. An amazing feeling of lightness started to accompany my runs. My breathing slowed, my legs stopped aching, and my body seemed to drift over the sand. Nina and I worked our way up to four miles and we ran that every single morning. Within four months, I had dropped 35 pounds and had gotten to the point where four miles felt easy. I wondered how much farther I could go. On the weekends, I started testing myself. Five miles, six miles, seven miles--good God, when I got to seven miles it was like the universe had opened up! At 37 years old, I was reborn. I seemed to have found my calling, my groove. I opened myself up to change and it led me to this amazing feeling that I could run forever if I just kept trying.

In an Olympic distance triathlon, you bike for 24.8 miles, swim about a mile, and then run a 10K. I had joined a triathlon training group and learned how to swim in open water. My running was on a roll. As for the bike, well, I figured I'd wing it. I rented a bicycle for race weekend and trusted I was in good enough shape that I could make it through.

The race began in Venice Beach just over a mile from my apartment, traveled through Hollywood and finished at the Staples Center in Downtown LA. Race morning felt beautiful. It was cool with a warm breeze--perfect conditions for racing. I figured at least 2,500 other athletes were competing, and I was shocked by the number of fit people around me. I struggled with some amount of nervousness, but I felt really, truly amazed that I was about to do something major in my life. I knew I had the swim and run down, but the bike--I was worried. Then my pal Nina—the one who challenged me to sign up in the first place--showed up.

"Hey Julie! You ready?"

"Are you ready?"

She was wearing flip flops. She strolled up to the crowd, walking her beach cruiser alongside her. It had a basket. She looked ready to go to the beach, not run a triathlon.

"Oh yeah," she said. "This is going to be a blast."

She had no cares about how she would do in the event, or how she looked. She didn't mind the very professional, very serious looking athletes staring at her as she placed the basket bike in the corral. I let my shoulders relax and took a deep breath. Now I knew there was a strong possibility that I wouldn't finish dead last.

At last, we lined up on the beach and got ready to swim. I hit the water with determination. All around me, other racers were freestyling their way through the waves. I felt a part of something bigger than myself and I felt a sense of camaraderie with everyone near me. Waves swelled and crashed, and I kept moving forward against the tide. After the first few meters, I tuned everything else out. The rest of the race was a blur. It was hard, sure. But that didn't register as I made my way to the finish chute. I was overjoyed and with the final steps I felt my arms begin to raise up, over my head.

I don't know if I thought that's what you were supposed to do at the end of the race, or if was just a spontaneous reaction to the joy I felt, but I took it all in with my outstretched arms. It was me, extending my power up to the sun! And that was where the Goddess pose was born. It felt good, crossing the line with my arms overhead, and I've done it in every race since (and later queened myself the Marathon Goddess, in part because of my trademark pose.)

I finished, well ahead of many other triathletes. But that didn't matter because I was just ecstatic that I had finished. It was time for a new challenge, so within hours, I signed up for a local half marathon in December, less than a month away.

I called my dad, of course. I told him about the tri and about the upcoming half marathon.

"Thirteen miles?" He asked in disbelief. It was a lot farther than a quarter-mile on the beach where I had started. "Julie, this is great. Keep going. I'll be cheering you on."

My dad kept his promise to cheer me on at my first half marathon. He was at the finish line armed with a camera. As I ran by during the last stretch, I saw him standing tall above the crowd, his body leaning over the barriers as he yelled at me to get to the finish line.

"There she is!" He bellowed. "There she is! Good job, Julie!"

When I finished, the first thought I had was: I could do that again. My dad was never really a hugger, but he gave me a solid pat on the back. I looked up at his eyes and told him I was going to do a marathon.

From that point on, so many of my conversations with my

dad were about running. He had a friend, he told me, who was part of this big group: the L.A. Road Runners, that rowdy group I saw on the beach just a year before—the people who were so fit it made me sad. They trained together, did their long runs together, and stuck in packs to do the L.A. Marathon. He urged me to give the club a shot. Immediately, I looked up the race date.

The race was in March 2008 a little over three months away. I had 13 miles under my belt already, and it would just be two of those, right? Why not try it? I looked up the L.A. Road Runners and searched for where to meet the Saturday morning group runs. I wondered if I would truly fit in, if there was anything special I needed to do to be a real runner. When I found the location, I realized that these were the same runners that had made me cry during my depressed days. Just to be part of them, even for one run, would be a beautiful thing.

So I suited up the very next Saturday. I had what I thought I needed: old sneakers and a gray, cotton sweat suit, like I was Rocky or something. I found someone with all the L.A. Road Runners gear on and asked her where I was supposed to go.

"What pace do you run at?"

I wasn't sure. I didn't have a watch. I ran however fast and far I felt like and figured out the mileage later, using maps or my car.

"I don't really know," I said. "I just ran a half marathon?" My voice shook a little bit and ended with the sort of upward inflection that means, "I don't really know what I'm doing here. Maybe I should just go home."

"Oh, that's perfect," she said. "What was your time?"

I told her it was a few minutes over two hours and that now I wanted to run a marathon. She brought me over to Group 5, which ran at a pace that, projected out to 26.2 miles, would result in a four-hour, ten-minute finish time. They trained at about a 10:45 or 11-minute per mile pace and she assured me that should be easy for me. There were introductions and welcomes. It felt intense, like I just enlisted myself into the Army and had this pressure to keep up or I would be stepped on and trampled over. I had no idea what I was doing.

I was in the pack of runners I had once admired. They were dressed lighter than me--shorts and neon jackets, new shoes, backpacks holding waters, and little belts that looked like fanny packs. The faint smell of body odor hovered over the group and I smiled. Sweat was just a part of this whole thing and no one was judging anyone here. I pulled my hair up in a ponytail and watched as the others did some stretches. And finally, we started running. The group asked me a lot of questions. Where did I train, what races had I done, what was I training for now? When I told them, I wanted to run the marathon in a month, they laughed--but not in a cruel way. They understood. I had that momentum and this new obsession, why not go for the big one?

"Just take it slow," one man said.

"And run with us every Saturday until the race," another said.

"And on race day, maybe don't wear all cotton."

Everyone laughed. I laughed, too. My sweat suit had been soaked through since mile 9, and I understood now that lighter clothing might be necessary. But these people believed in me, and I believed I could do it, too. I was going to run a damn marathon. I couldn't wait to tell everyone.

"Remember my name," I said. March 2, 2008 finally arrived and it was time for me to run my first marathon. I was only kidding around, but I felt like there was some truth behind it. It was race morning, and I was on the bus with the other marathoners getting shuttled to the start line of the L.A. Marathon from Universal. I turned to look at the passengers across from me with my long legs spilling into the aisle. The dark navy-blue morning sky made us all shadows. I couldn't help myself, this energy charged through me--half adrenaline, half genuine giddiness. I felt like I was on the verge of some magic transcendence.

"It's my first marathon," I told the other people on the bus. "I think I'm going to break four hours. Hell, I might even qualify for Boston!"

I didn't even know what that meant. I had just heard that was something people tried to do at marathons. The people around me laughed and clapped.

It had been a whirlwind of a morning already. I woke up, got dressed in a random assortment of old stuff, including--for some reason-- a baseball hat. I had never trained in a hat before, but I was under the impression that a hat was required to run a marathon and so on it went. I ran out of the house and got in the car. I didn't realize, of course, that the marathon would close my local roads and so I circled around to find parking like a crazy woman, white knuckling the steering wheel, praying I would be able to find my pace group before the race. I sprinted to the shuttle location. That pre-race anxiety is a real thing, but once I got on the bus, I melted into the seat and felt the excitement start to build inside me.

Another passenger told someone behind us that I was running my first marathon.

"L.A. is a great first marathon," he said. "Good luck,

you're going to do great."

"I'm so ready," I said. "Maybe I'll win this thing!"

Chatting with strangers about running was second nature to me now. I felt so welcomed by this group and I knew most of them didn't believe that I would break four hours or run a Boston qualifying time, but everyone around me wished me luck. Experienced runners told me course secrets, newer runners shared their fears and I could relate. Would I finish? Of course, I figured.

I've got this.

And for the first 11 miles I did have it. I was flying. I ran past people, smiling and waving, telling them all I was going to break four hours. And then, it hit. The Wall I had heard so much about Except it wasn't supposed to be happening this early in the race.

Now, in hindsight, I recognize that the blazing pace I went out in might've been my ruination. But on that day, I just kept thinking, what the hell is going on with me? My legs started feeling heavy and my pace slowed. I struggled through three more miles and realized I had 14.2 more to go. Walking hurt just as bad as running, so I kept trucking on in a half-run, with my new watch reading 10-minute miles, then 11-minute miles. I was hobbling. I ignored water stations. I watched other runners eating small gummy things and wondered what on earth they were doing. Was I supposed to be doing that too? I could smell my own sweat and I wanted to hurl.

My ex-husband Frank had come to mile 18 to cheer me on and I saw him standing in the crowd. I wanted to wave but I couldn't. He was looking right at me with a concerned look on his face. He wasn't waving or cheering. I made my way to his side of the course very slowly.

"Julie!" He finally said. "Is that you?"

I couldn't speak.

"OK. OK, girl. Just a little bit more," he said. "You need water? You might need water. You OK, though?"

I nodded. He looked worried.

"You know," he said. "I tried to get the kids to come, but I don't think they understand how big this is." Frank held a flimsy piece of poster board with the words, "Go Julie" scribbled in his lopsided handwriting. It felt wonderful to have someone there, and to have Frank, who had seen me at my worst, so genuinely proud of me. I wanted to assure him that I understood why they didn't want to come. They were teens after all. But I couldn't form words. I just drank water and nodded.

"They are going to be damn proud of you," he said.

That little pick-me-up from Frank, the most unlikely source, truly kept me going. I even tried to pick it up a little bit as I continued away from him, but there was nothing in me. I could feel my shoulders curl down and my head felt heavy. Finally, what felt like ten years later, I saw the finish. I made it. My time? Four hours, 40 minutes. I barely made it to the last timing mat before I sat down. Later Frank would tell me that he was concerned I might just die in front of him. I shook my head and looked at my watch.

"I feel like hell," I said. "I'm never doing that again."

Chapter 6
A Second
Chance with Papa

I ran my next marathon three months later and it went slightly better than the first. I still didn't know what I was doing, but as many runners do, I felt like I needed redemption. And I kept finding little gems in this running scene: friends in the LA Road Runners, a new sense of self and purpose, a slimmer waistline, and goals—both personal and universal.

One thing I couldn't stop hearing about from the runners around me was Boston. Finally, I asked a member of my pace group about it.

She explained that the Boston Marathon, run April of every

year, was the race everyone wanted to run. It started in 1897, and
it is the oldest and most prestigious marathon in the world, outside
of the Olympics. But besides its long and heralded history, it has
an important distinction few other marathons have: You need to
demonstrate a certain level of competency to run it. Unlike most
other major marathons, from New York to Chicago, running Boston is not just a question of paying to register. In Boston, each age
group has a qualifying time that needs to be met prior to your en-
try. In other words, I learned, you couldn't just sign up and go run
26.2—you had to be fast. For my age group at the time, I would
have to run a 3:50; almost an hour faster than my first marathon!
But when I broke it down, that came out to about an 8:30 per mile
pace. I could do that, I thought. I was running almost every mile at
about a 9-minute pace, so I figured I could knock off 30 seconds,
no problem. I was new to this running thing, with lots of room
for improvement. I'd come so far already, going from gasping for
breath and falling in the sand, to several full marathons, albeit at a
much slower time than 3:50.

"I'm going to do that," I declared to my pace group as we
jogged along. "I'm going to qualify for Boston." Running had bol-
stered my optimism and positive thinking. Of course, I didn't realize that running a faster marathon required a careful training for-

mula designed to acclimate your leg and cardiovascular muscles to a quicker pace over such a long distance. I still didn't know anything about fueling and nutrition.

And while I had now acquired some healthy new habits, it takes a long time to truly shed the layers you build up around you. For me, those layers included my unwillingness to ask for help, even in this venture. I just figured that if I kept running the distance, I'd get faster by some sort of marathon magic.

After that training run, I gave my dad a call. He was always the first person I wanted to talk to after a good run and when I had a new, bright idea.

"Papa," I said. I was still panting, drenched in sweat and too excited to slow my breathing.

"Hi Julie," he said.

"Have you heard about the Boston Marathon?"

"I think I know something about it," he replied.

"You have to qualify to get in. I need to run a 3:50," I said. I could just picture him doing some quick calculations in his head.

"You haven't run under four hours yet," he said.

"I've got this," I told him.

"OK, then!" he said. I could tell he was pumped. Sure, he was thrilled that I was getting in shape and running every day, but my dad had a hunger for competition. With his long-burning desire to have a son to root for in any sport, my newfound passion was at last filling that void in his life. Now not only was I running, I was running towards being a member of the accomplished runners who make it into Boston. Papa was also in awe of the distance—he knew getting through 26.2 miles is not something just anyone can do. Hell, he couldn't do it, even in his prime. He was always drawn to quick spurts of movement and enjoyed time on the tennis or racquetball court. He'd taken a few classes at the local gym and swam and kept his body moving, but running more than a mile at a time was just not in his blood. His admiration for my stamina, hard work, and patience made me feel like I was a varsity athlete.

Our conversations about running slowly mended the years of turmoil our relationship had gone through. I remember another call after a run one evening.

"Hey Papa," I said.

"Julie!" Even though we lived less than 10 minutes away from each other and had dinner every week, every time I called him was like a celebration. He now seemed to love hearing my voice, and I loved to hear his; a stark change from a year or so earlier, when he couldn't seem to stand the sight of me. I asked about his day.

"How's your running?" He said.

"Well that's why I called," I told him. "I fought with myself all day. I needed to do 10 miles. That's what was on the plan. And I just kept putting it off. I was like really fighting with myself."

"That happens," he said.

"Yeah, but I sucked it up and I put on my running shoes, and I just walked down to the pier and I started. And I was so happy I did. The sun was setting and the whole sky just opened into all these colors. Papa, if you saw the sun out there, you would've fainted."

"Julie, good for you. I mean it, that's true beauty right there," he said.

His snide remarks about my poor eating and weight disappeared. He no longer criticized me for life decisions that I couldn't change. We didn't have some beautiful, heartfelt moment of reckoning, we just enjoyed each other and talked—really talked—more often. Now I know that he was most proud that I was doing something for myself, something that was really making me happy.

For some people, running is a part of their life. For me, running became my entire life. In 2009, I was running nonstop, a different marathon each month with group runs and shorter races in between.

The marathons were going well, but not surprisingly, I still wasn't seeing the results I wanted. At every marathon, when I would hit the final stretch, I'd look up at the time and see the glaring red numbers taunting me: Four hours and change. I really didn't know what I was doing wrong—but it's not like I was changing anything in my training or race preparations or strategy either and it was my old stubbornness that prevented me from seeking help or listening to some of the sound advice of other runners.

During group runs with the L.A. Road Runners, I loved chatting, but I hated when people mentioned that my form was off or that I wasn't doing enough speed work. I liked to run at one pace. Running was my joy and running faster would require more effort. Why would I want to make it harder? Besides, I didn't want to be prescribed a fix from someone because running was my thing. I truly thought the more marathons I ran, the faster I would get. I thought I was destined to do it and be great at it, all in good time.

Many races, I didn't wear a watch. I ran mostly by feel, locking into the same pace that I trained at, and I never thought that was a bad thing. Members of my training group encouraged me to reach out to a coach. There was one guy—a master of the craft who would be sure to help me reach my goal. David Levine. He was the race director for the City of Angels Half Marathon and served as a pace leader for the Road Runners. And he was a coach par excellence. On his website, he promised to get any runner to reach their true potential. This was going to be my guy. After one group run, I thought about going over and introducing myself. I'd seen him before in passing and knew who this legend was. But when I went over to introduce myself, he looked busy, calming down an overexcited man who appeared to be having a nervous breakdown because he'd fallen off his pace group.

I listened closely to David soothing this overwrought guy.

"I just... I thought I was in good shape and my race is just three weeks away, and I couldn't even run my training pace?" said the runner.

"Jerry, it's warm today," David said with such gentleness. "What did you eat last night?"

"A burger."

"What did you drink?"

"Water."

"What else?"

"Beer."

"Ah! And did you sleep well?"

"Not really."

"Perhaps work is stressing you out?"

"Okay, yeah, it hasn't been my week."

"So this is not an issue. You still got your miles in, and once you stopped fighting yourself, your heart rate went down. Run slower for all your easy runs this week and take in some electrolytes, okay?"

He gave Jerry a hearty pat on the back. Other exhausted and frantic looking runners engulfed him, each with their own concerns and anxieties. I began to wonder if this guy Levine was really a psychologist.

I started to have second thoughts. I needed a coach, not a therapist. Besides, I didn't want to beg. I wasn't going to wait in line to ask him how to run a marathon—I was doing just fine getting through the 26.2 on my own. I just had to figure out how to move a little faster. I figured I'd have a breakthrough at one of my next races.

The running community swallowed me whole, and I was tuned in to all the latest happenings in the SoCal circuit. Word on the running street was that the L.A. Marathon was thinking about changing its course for the upcoming year. The original route took you from Universal City to downtown, basically through an industrial area and Skid Row. The proposed change would lead runners through my home turf—along the beaches of Santa Monica. I wanted this change so bad, it became an obsession for me. I wanted to make the course change a reality, not just for me, but for the thousands of other runners who would run the race.

I heard there was going to be a meeting at Santa Monica City Hall about the change and I decided to go. I'd never been to an open forum like this and I wasn't even sure what I was doing there. The old building was art deco style and loomed over Main Street. As I entered into the auditorium space, I saw about 25 runners or so there about the marathon course. In total there were probably 100 people including councilmen behind desks, on stage, looking very important. I had signed up earlier in the week to be one of the speakers and share my thoughts. I had never done anything like this before. When they called me up, I was terrified. Seeing all the faces turned to look at me, I broke into a sweat. The hairs on my arms raised, my hands shook.

"Shit," I thought. "What am I doing?" I'd never spoken in public before. I was a mom and an accountant, not a spokeswoman.

I took the microphone.

"Hi," I said. My voice shook. Get it together, what are you

going to say? I thought.

"Hi," I started over with a little more authority now. "My name is Julie, and I just wanted to speak on behalf of the runners. I haven't been running long, but LA was my first race. Right now, this year, I've run 10 marathons so far…"

A few people clapped. Ok, I thought, they get it.

"I just thought I'd let you guys on the city council know that what you're proposing, the altered route, would be such a huge improvement to the course. Nobody coming to LA wants to see Skid Row. If they're anything like me, just a normal runner looking for a beautiful race, they want to run along the beaches. They want to smell the water, not the city. This could be a really big deal for our race, for both the people who call LA home and the thousands of runners who visit us to run our course."

There, I did it. It was all a blur after I spoke. I don't remember if anyone commented or if anybody clapped. I sank into my chair, relieved. In the audience, I saw some of the big players: the legendary Coach Levine, another coach, and other members of the L.A. Road Runners board. Out of the corner of my eye, I saw the club's administrator lean into David and whisper something.

After the meeting, I was standing outside with another local coach, Bill Lockton, who I knew well. It was a warm July night. I was wearing my favorite white miniskirt and a black blouse, and now, after my speech, feeling like a rock star. David approached me, and Bill introduced us.

"Glad to make it official," David said. "I've seen you running."

"Yeah," I said. "I think we've said hi a few times."

"Yeah, that's usually the best I can come up with."

He moved and talked quickly, like he was running even when he was standing still. He slid his glasses up on his nose and squinted into the sun. "Thanks for what you said in there. You know, we were impressed. Would you ever consider being a pace leader?"

"For the Road Runners?"

"Yeah," he said. "The powers that be said I should do whatever I could to get you to lead a group, so what is it going to take?" He grinned. "How about a t shirt?"

"OK," I said, playing it cool. I wanted to jump in his arms and say yes! Yes, of course I will lead runners, this is what I now live for. But instead, I tried to play hard to get. "I'm trying to qualify for Boston right now, so maybe the next training cycle."

Other runners joined our little pack in the parking lot and we chatted as the sun went down. The words of the other runners floated around me and I listened and nodded. Some people asked about my races, and what I had next on the calendar. Around me, there was talk of shoes and electrolytes and track workouts and I smiled easily and nodded, not so much understanding everything that was being said, but just enjoying the moment. I felt involved and embraced and that I had found somewhere in the world where I truly belonged.

I had too many races on my calendar to count. A half marathon one weekend, and a marathon the next Sunday. This is not a good running life. I was falling into a common trap of overuse and over-racing, like a lot of new runners. At the 2010 L.A. Marathon, the first on the new course, which they labeled "Stadium to the Sea," I spotted my dad at mile 14. Again, his broad shoulders and all 230-lbs of him spilled over onto the race course as he cheered.

"There she is!" He boomed.

He held out coconut water for me to drink, while filming me with his video camera. "Thanks, Papa," I said. "But I have to run!" I felt his pride wrap around me. Of course, I had another marathon right around the corner. I was addicted to the distance and addicted to the positive attention I finally earned from my father. But I still couldn't crack the four-hour barrier. I promised myself that this next race—number 17—I would break four and maybe even qualify for Boston.

But I finally admitted to myself that the only way I was going to reach that goal was by asking for help. Maybe I was running too much or not running right at all. I loved that my 12 marathons in 12 months had gotten me inducted into the Marathon Maniacs, a national group of bona fide running-crazies, but all my marathons weren't getting me to where I wanted to go: Boston.

It was time for a new approach. I e-mailed David and asked him to make me a plan. I told him how determined I was to hit this goal. A day or so later, he e-mailed me back. Sorry, he said, he was busy writing "The Complete Idiot's Guide to Marathon Training" and didn't have time to take on a new athlete.

"Nope," I said to the computer screen. I needed help and I wasn't about to wait for the release of "The Idiot's Guide" to get this guy to help me to the finish. I called a friend and asked if she would join me for a track workout that week with the Road Runners. I'd never stepped foot on a track before, but I knew David would be there. It's easy to say no over e-mail, but if I just showed up and went through a few laps, he'd understand I meant business. Besides, he was supposedly recruiting me to be a pace leader— he would recall our conversation from the town hall meeting. Or maybe he'd remember me as the bronzed, long-haired woman in the bikini top out on the boardwalk during every group run.

The track smelled like burnt rubber. The sun seemed to bounce off it, radiating heat and smoldering through my worn shoes. Other runners looked like they'd been going for miles already. They breezed around the track talking to one another, bursting into high knees and butt kicks and long skips. David stood near a line in the middle of one of the track's long stretches. I recognized his glasses and blue L.A. Running Club jacket. My girlfriend and I dropped our stuff near the bleachers and walked towards him.

"Welcome, you're just in time," he said with a smile. I caught his eye and knew right away that he was totally checking me out. I figured he must've recognized me now from the meeting and maybe connected my face to my name. I smiled back at him, but I wasn't feeling a magnetic attraction. No, to me, David Levine looked like a total running nerd. His clean-cut and kind demeanor stood in stark comparison to my type: the rough and tumble bad dudes. Ditch those nerdy glasses and get a skull and crossbones tattoo on that chicken leg and maybe I'd reconsider. But I didn't mind the extra attention. And hey, maybe a little bit of flirtation could get me my marathon plan.

"Do you ladies need to warm up or are you ready to go?"

We shook our heads no, incredulous at this suggestion. A running warm up for more running?

I used my first mile to get warm, no matter what the distance. To my left and right, runners dripping in sweat were lining up. Men who smelled like cologne and dirty laundry stepped in front of me right on the white line next to David. I drifted to the back.

"OK everyone," David yelled to the crowd. "Let's start with a 400, nice and easy. Then we'll launch into an 800 at about 80 percent effort."

With that, his hand went down, and everyone took off. After a beat, I started pumping my legs. The pack charged forward, leaving me behind after just a few strides. How was this nice and easy? And how long was a 400 anyway? I don't think I'd ever run faster than my standard 9-minute pace. I ran everything there in what I felt was my sweet spot. Now, I was running in a circle, just trying to chase down a group of people who had already stopped on the line and were preparing to take off again.

When I finally made it back around, David smiled and told me to just try and push on. "Two times around this time," he said with that sweet smile. I was breathing hard, trying to work spit out of my mouth. I couldn't return the smile this time. I was already dreading the next lap. "This should be a nice, hard effort. Just try to run how you just did and try to be consistent. Ready?"

Some of the faster runners were coming around already. I nodded my head.

"OK. Go!"

My legs felt like lead. My arms flailed at my sides. I gasped for each breath and knew that this wasn't 80 percent effort, this was 100 percent and yet it was still so slow. Runners blew by me and I kept chugging along, taking every painful step and wishing it were my last. Why was this so hard? Around the second curve of the track, I started letting off the gas, sinking into a sloppy jog. My throat hurt, my chest ached, and my salad from lunch started spinning around in my stomach. I half-jogged down the straightaway back to where David stood.

"Let's stop there for today," he said.

I bent over, with my hands on my knees and stared down at the red rubber of the track.

"I don't like this," I said, gasping.

David laughed. After just a half-mile, my workout was done. I waited for Tammy to finish (she hadn't fared much better) and we collected our stuff.

"You can't leave yet," David said. "You have to at least stay to hear my joke," he said.

All the runners gathered around him and broke into synchronized stretches that David called and counted out. We followed along. When he got to a seated inner thigh stretch, which involves using your elbows to gently press down on your inner thigh muscles as you hold on to your ankles or toes, the other runners started laughing before David even had a chance to open his mouth.

"Okay, now almost everyone knows this by now," he said. "But go down and hold for the next several seconds. And if you hear a loud tearing noise, you've just injured yourself."

The other runners erupted with groans and applause and laughter. A woman turned to me and Tammy and explained that David had just told the joke.

"That was it? The joke?" Tammy said.

The runner said he said the same thing, at the same time, every practice. It wasn't funny. And yet, it was. I laughed along. Maybe track wasn't that bad.

Even though my grand plan to show David just how determined I was had failed, I got to see this man in his element. I had a lot of respect for what he did, even if his joke was terrible. Since

I'd nearly thrown up on his shoes, I didn't think I was looking cute enough to flirt my way into getting a coach, so I stumbled away from practice as quickly as possible. But at the next group run, I saw him again and things had changed.

"Julie!" he said. "Hey, you know, I have a little bit of free time. Are you still interested in that training schedule?"

I was ecstatic. Perhaps he saw just what a mess I was, and how I didn't know what I was doing, and took pity on me. Or maybe he liked me, but at that moment I didn't care. I was happy to have him on my side. We planned a run together where he would hang with me and listen to my breath and watch my stride.

We started at the totem pole in Santa Monica. It's on the corner of Ocean Avenue and San Vicente, which happens to be about mile 25 of the L.A Marathon. It was the perfect day to run, with a little breeze and the sweet scent of the ocean cooling everything down. David's attention was completely and totally on me, and I loved it. I thought it was pretty cool to be treated kind of like a test subject. I wondered if he'd find the cure to all my running woes and be able to fix me on the spot. I thought maybe it had something to do with my stride, that my left leg kicked out to the side too much, or that I simply wasn't pushing myself hard enough.

"The point of this run is for me to hear your breathing," he said. I nodded at this seemingly odd request. "We have to figure out what pace you need to train at and what pace will keep your heart rate low enough to get maximum benefits on your easy days," he explained. "Do you know what pace you're running on your easy days?"

I ran my easy days the same way I ran my races. My plan to that point was one pace fits all.

"That's what I thought," he said after I didn't answer. "Rookie mistake. Everyone thinks they should be running fast all the time. OK break's over, let's run."

I thought he might really put me through the paces, really test my aerobic capacity. The first mile felt easy and enjoyable. I liked being with David and I liked running next to him on a dirt path above Ocean Avenue. I tried to speed up a little bit, wanting to impress him on our first training date, but he hung back, forcing me to maintain a slow pace. He listened carefully to the rhythm of my breath and then, inexplicably, told me to walk.

"Walk? Why?"

He smiled in his very gentle way.

"Oh, Julie," he said, teasing me a little. "Just trust me."

So, I walked. My hands on my hips, the sweat pooling on

my forehead.

He kept asking me what my heart rate was, like every two minutes. We would run. Then we would walk. This jog-walk non-sense continued on for what felt like forever. This wasn't running, I wanted to yell at him. This isn't fun. Didn't he understand that I liked running because of the freedom it brought. If I stopped and walked, the entire point would be lost. Yet I did trust him, and I liked him.

He had a true kindness in his eyes. But all that changed when I got the training plan. I called him immediately.

"David. What is all this 11-minute pace stuff?"

Every easy run—and there were a lot of easy runs—was supposed to be 11-minute mile pace. Then, mixed in, were dreaded track days. Very rarely would I get to run at my happy 9-minute pace.

"This better fucking work."

He laughed. "Julie, I always say when you get to the point where you're swearing at me, that means you're doing it right. I want you to go slow."

I went slow. I plodded along the beach and on the streets, racking up more and more miles in terribly sluggish times. I'd check in with David on track days and tell him I was swearing at him for every single mile I was forced to go at that miserable pace. But I felt OK, good even. And on those speed days, I would die, but I would make it through. And then, something miraculous started to happen. Tempo paces started feeling easier. I could keep up with the pack during track intervals. Holding an 8:20 pace for six miles, something that would've seemed impossible during my 12 marathons in 12 months, felt incredibly easy. And hey, I would only have to do that for 20 more miles.

On my 20-miler, David broke out his dorkiest helmet and bike and rode alongside me. I tried going faster, again, to impress him and show him how far I had come. But he scolded me and told me to slow down, these 20 miles would be the toughest in the training plan and the miles that would most prepare me to race. He handed me a drink—his secret and special concoction of electrolytes and vitamins—that kept my energy up. I slobbered its citrusy contents all over myself as I ran, still not mastering the drinking-while-running skill so many other marathoners seemed to have down. We agreed that if the drink settled in my stomach, I would use it for the rest of my long training runs and on race day. I was all in.

When we were done, I didn't feel destroyed. I gave him a hug.

"I think it's working," I said. "But we'll see."

"It is working, Julie," he said. "I know you can do it. Boston, watch out."

I stuck to the plan, crossing out every workout as I completed it. Every long run, I called my dad. Every track workout, I called my dad.

"What's the coach making you do this week?"

"Ugh, still making me run slow."

"And then fast on the track?"

"Yup, still the same game plan."

"Do you think it's working?"

"I don't know yet, but he's coached a lot of people who stuck to the plan and then really made it."

"What's he like?"

"What do you mean, Papa?"

"Is he a good guy?"

I laughed. I knew what my dad might be up to. I thought that maybe he was trying to hook me up with a "nice runner."

"He's a great guy, he's really sweet."

"Good."

He would encourage me when I sounded ragged and cheer when I hit a new distance. On the day of my 20-miler, he and my mom were on a trip in Australia, and while I was sad I couldn't call him to tell him about the success, I was happy he was out doing what he loved. But they came home the next day, much earlier than expected. My mom called—and said he wasn't feeling well.

"He's just not himself right now," she said.

"What does that mean, though?" I knew he had been having some heartburn and my mom had told me he'd been more tired than usual. But to leave a trip early? Something must've been really bothering him.

"It's his stomach," she said. "I think he has really bad indigestion. You know how bad heartburn can make you feel."

"Well, are you going to the doctor?"

"Yes"

"Good. Keep me posted."

I started thinking of him in the past few weeks. He'd lost weight, but he was happy about that. My dad was a guy who loved his food, so when he started to shed some weight without changing his diet, he thought it was a dream come true. But I remembered seeing him coming home from the gym one night before their trip to Australia. He looked frail in a way he never had before.

"Papa, are you okay?" I had asked him.

"Never better!" he responded confidently.

After his visit to his physician, I went over to their house to find out what was going on. In the old living room with the piano, we all sat down together and I braced myself for something.

"What did the doctor say, dad?"

"Acid reflux," he said. "I'm gonna be around for another 20 years! Sorry!"

I laughed, but one glance at my mother told me she was still worried. It just wasn't quite right. I shrugged her concern off for the moment, just happy that he was happy and that there wasn't too much cause for worry. I told him about the 20-miler with David and that my goal race, The Long Beach Marathon, was just a few weeks away.

"Are you ready?" He asked.

"I think so," I said. "This time, Papa, I'm gonna BQ." I had no question that Long Beach would be the marathon where I would finally do it. I'd trained perfectly, had a few supporters on the course, had my special electrolyte formula from David, and I was ready to roll. I hadn't slept well and I had no real race plan, but that didn't matter.

I coasted along for the first six miles, going at a conservative pace that felt easy to my legs. Just past the mile marker, I spotted Rod Dixon, the coach of the L.A. Road Runners. Rod was a stud—a very handsome man who'd won The New York City

Marathon in 1983. I had a little crush on him and I knew I needed to stop and say hi.

"Rod!" I ran up to him with outstretched arms. We embraced.

"You're looking great, Julie," he said in his adorable New Zealand accent.

"I feel great," I said, "This is going to be my race."

I saw him again at mile 15 and I still felt great, which was unbelievable to me. I felt no signs of fatigue and thought I could run the pace I was at for another 11 miles with ease.

"Rod!" I shouted again. I gave him another hug. "Can I pick it up now?"

"Not yet," he said, with a big smile. "Keep it smooth."

I fell back into my cadence and kept going along. David was at mile 20 with a grin on his face.

"Way to go, Julie!" I couldn't help it, I gave him a hug too. I was so happy to see him and I wanted to thank him for all the work he had put into my marathon plan, and how he had completely changed my perception of proper training. I wanted to say all of this, but I knew I had to finish the race first. Just six more miles to go, and I was still feeling amazing. When my watch beeped at mile 23, I knew I only had 3.2 miles left, but when I looked at my time, I saw that I was cutting it close—too close. I tried to do quick math. In order to still make it under the qualifying time, I was going to have to run 8-minute miles for a little over three miles.

"Shit," I thought as I stomped down the road. "Shit, shit, shit."

I swore with every step, trying to kick my legs into high gear. I didn't think I could do it. Where had the time gone? How could I feel so good, have everything go right, and still not make it? Was it all that hugging that had cost me precious time?

I ran my heart out in those last miles, trying my best to get my worn legs to move. But when I saw the race clock, I got nervous. I reminded myself that the race clock wasn't the right time. My watch said 3:50.

Maybe, just maybe, I had made it.

I called my dad. I wanted him to be proud of me. I thought maybe there was a chance I did it and the clocks were wrong. I left him a message.

"Papa," I said. "I think I did it. I think we're going to Boston."

It was kind of a lie, because I wasn't sure yet.

I stuffed my phone into my finisher's bag and tried to get away from the race as quickly as possible.

I was able to log on to the results after the race in my hotel room. The official timers clocked me at 3:52. Two minutes over the qualifying time. The hugs. The hugs cost me my BQ.

I even sent the Long Beach Marathon an e-mail to ask if their clocks were wrong, but to no avail. I offered to show them my Garmin, but it wasn't going to work.

I was in some sort of marathon denial. I'd told so many people, I trained so hard, I put everything I had into this race—to come up short shattered my world.

But it was true. There was no timing glitch. It wasn't a typo. I had run a 3:52, plain and simple. My dad had called my cell to congratulate me, and when I called him back, I had to tell him that it wasn't true. I was close, but I hadn't made it in on time.

"But you broke four hours," he said with genuine excitement in his voice. "One goal out of two, Julie. You're gonna do it next time."

Chapter 7
A Devastating Loss

I woke the next morning and rolled back over, covering my head with the blanket. My legs ached. My heart ached. I had worked so hard—all those slow miles and track workouts and special electrolyte drinks— and I was still minutes off a Boston qualifying time. I replayed the race in my head, mile after mile, trying to figure out what I'd done. Was it the hugs? A slow start?

I'd told everyone I was going to qualify for Boston, and now I felt like a disappointment not only to myself, but to them. My dad especially. Despite his supportive reaction, I wanted him to be able to say that his daughter was part of an elite class of marathoners. I already had a redemption race on the calendar: Sacramento in December, just two months away. I stretched each muscle while laying down, thinking of the training I still had to do. My phone buzzed; my mother was calling.

"Hello," I answered. My voice sounded hoarse and tired.

"Julie," she sounded even worse than me.

"What's wrong, mom?"

"Julie, I've got news and it's not good," she said. I braced myself.

"It's Papa," she said.

"What? What is it?"

There was a long pause, she was searching for the right way to say it, I'm sure.

"He's got pancreatic cancer, stage four, and there is nothing they can do."

Everything turned gray. The light from my windows darkened, shadows grew up the walls in my room. She must be wrong. Blood rushed to my head and all I could think was that this was a mistake, a bad diagnosis, perhaps the result of an overly zealous doctor.

There was no way my father would have cancer that was so advanced. He'd been to the doctor. They said he was fine. They'd said it was reflux. A chill ran up and down my back, each vertebra vibrating, a cold sweat dripping down from my neck. I told her I would be right over, and I stumbled out of bed into my car. I pulled up to my parents' home and tried to breathe. I knew I had to be strong and rational. They were shaken, and they needed positivity and hope. I held my breath for a moment and closed my eyes and tried to picture light. I wanted to bring that glow into the house with me and shine it onto my dad. He needed me now.

I walked in the front door.

"Hello?"

It felt smaller inside than it had before. A thin layer of dust covered the piano.

"Mom?"

I rounded the corners, walking from room to room. My father was in his bed with my mom sitting next to him. She leapt up and I embraced her. Then I leaned down to my dad and kissed his cheek. I didn't know what to say. Accusing them of not being right about the cancer seemed silly now with him huddled under blankets. He looked small and pale, but he was awake. I could feel denial leaving my system and I knew I would have to tell him the most cliché thing any cancer patient has ever heard, but it was what felt true to my heart in that moment.

"We're going to beat this," I said.

My mom looked at me with shock written across her face.

"But Julie, they said…" she started.

I put a hand up and shook my head.

"No," I said. "Papa, I know what they said. But nothing is impossible. I know how strong you are. You know how strong you are. Let's keep going as long as we can."

His face brightened a little. The doctors had given him a death sentence, saying he only had six months. I couldn't bear to think like that. No one could know for sure how much time he had. I wanted him, no matter how bad it was, to have some hope, to feel somewhat normal, to feel like he had us on his side.

"Let's keep being positive," I said. "We still have lots of time."

He smiled. My mom cried. I wrapped an arm around her and we stayed quiet for a little while.

My sister came shortly after. We stayed in his room and sat together until my dad drifted to sleep. The three of us then went to the kitchen to talk. There wasn't much to say other than what the doctors had told my mom, but I made her recount every detail. It was grim. He would be in a lot of pain. The cancer would slowly take over and steal his appetite, his organs, and his life.

"What are they doing for it?" My sister asked. "What can we do?"

"Well, they said the only thing we can do is manage the pain," my mom said. "We have to keep him comfortable."

"So they're not treating it?" I said.

"No," said my mom. Tears clung to her bottom eyelashes. Her eyes were etched with red marks.

"Oh my god," my sister Diana said.

"No," I said. "He's going to beat it."

"But what if he doesn't?" Diana was pleading.

"Diana, don't talk like that," I said. "He is not going to die. He is going to beat this thing. You'll see!"

I didn't know what would happen if he didn't pull through. The pain in the house was unbearable. My mother, trying to be strong, turned away from us, started busying herself, unfolding and refolding a dish towel while looking out the kitchen window.

I started going through logical next steps: second opinions, specialty diets, clinical trials. But I knew first, before any proactive measures, I had to get them to believe in a miracle.

"Listen," I said, grabbing my sister's arm, "we have to believe that this is something we can all get through. We must believe that he can and will beat this. We just need time to figure out how."

My mom stood with her back to us, her shoulders quivering, her head down. I couldn't know her pain. This man, her husband, has been in her life for 52 years.

"Mom," I reached over to hug her. She fell into my arms. "We can do this. We all have to believe."

Just as I believed I was going to qualify for Boston, I felt certain my dad could beat this diagnosis.

The next day, my mom drove him to Cedars-Sinai Medical Center. The pain had taken a turn for the worse. The same day, she took herself to Santa Monica Hospital for a planned surgery to have her kidney removed. She had to get it done and in the midst of my father's diagnosis, didn't have enough time to reschedule. For a week, I was rushing back and forth between hospitals, making sure they were both OK, relaying messages from one to the other.

Day after day, I arrived thinking I would make it to his room and find him, maybe, better. Sitting up and talking with his usual energy. Eating and chatting with the nurses. But instead, his skin grew more yellow, hanging loosely over his bones.

Three days into his hospital stay, I armed myself with a toaster and made my way to his room. I looked down the halls to make sure no nurses were coming our way, crouched down and started looking for a power outlet.

"Julie," my dad said. He was drowsy from the pain medication. "What are you doing?"

I moved his IV stand out of the way and found what I was looking for. I placed the toaster on the chair I usually sat in, took out a bagel I had sliced back at my house, and placed it inside. The cold antiseptic hospital smell drifted out of the room and the air filled with the smell of warmed bread. I kept a close eye on the red coils and bagel, careful not to let it burn or start smoking. Bagels, a staple from his New York life, were my dad's favorite food. A true comfort.

I saw his eyes light up when he smelled the bagel toasting. He smiled.

"They just don't do bagels here," he said.

"Do you want butter or cream cheese?" I asked.

He waved his hand.

"Just dry?"

The bagel popped up and I put it on a plate for him. I took the butter and cream cheese from my bag and set it near the bed in case he changed his mind. I put the toaster on the floor in a hiding place behind a chair and sat down.

"How was your run?" he said. He held the bagel in his big hand, examining it.

"I didn't run today," I said. "Dad, how am I supposed to run with you in here?"

He tried to take a bite. It was a small piece. He chewed it over and over, slow and with care. I could tell that he was hungry for it—for a slice of normalcy. He swallowed with discomfort. But I could tell he had enjoyed it.

"You can't stop," he said. "Why wouldn't you run? You need to."

"OK, sure, I'll run tomorrow," I said, trying to placate him. For once, running was not the highest priority.

"No, Julie," he said. "I'm telling you. You have to work, you have to run, you have to keep living your life. That's what will help me the most. Don't do anything different on account of me. When is the next race?"

"It's in two months, about."

"So why take a day off?" he said. "Where is it anyway?"

"It's in Sacramento, Papa."

I didn't know what to say. Here was my father, the only man I'd ever wanted to please, sick in a hospital with a morphine drip and who'd eaten nothing but a morsel of bagel for the past four days, telling me that I better not stop running.

"Papa, you wanna go with me to the race?"

"Yes."

He wasn't kidding. He looked right at me and I knew what

he was asking for—he needed something to look forward to.

That night at home, I searched for plane tickets and hotels. Sitting in front of the computer, I felt myself relax in the familiar world of planning for a marathon. I knew my mom would think dad's plan to accompany me to my next race was a fever dream, but I didn't care. She didn't have to know. My dad is going to see me BQ, I thought. My dad is going to live and he is going to see me BQ. I repeated it over and over.

In the morning, I took Jessie out to do a quick run. Easy pace, nothing fancy, just a loop around the neighborhood. The hospital decided to release my dad, and I was ready to tell him about the race and our trip and get him home to rest up until he was well enough to get on the plane with me. I was excited to tell him I ran. It was for him, this time. All my miles, I would dedicate to his recovery.

Back home after the run, I told the kids to get ready. We were all going to bust Papa out of his hospital room. They looked scared. My son went into his room and shut the door.

"Everything is OK," I said to Samantha. "It's all going to be fine."

"Mother," she said, "I don't know. Ma is so scared. And last time we were over there, with grandpa in bed and stuff, it just felt different. Papa was talking about life and what a good life he's had. When I looked at Frankie, he was crying."

I took my daughter in my arms, still sweat-soaked from the run.

"Are you sure?" I said. I didn't know he was feeling this so deeply or that any of them thought differently than me. I figured my brave face and attitude would be enough to go on, and that they would find comfort in my optimism.

"I don't know," she said, crying into my shoulder. "I don't want to lose him."

"I know."

"But listen," I said, "there is nothing to cry about. It's all going to be fine. We're all going to go to Sacramento. Papa, too. He's beating this right now."

I was telling this to my daughter, but also myself. At the hospital, I'd seen a version of my father I'd never seen before. Having to bring him food, seeing nurses tend to him, witnessing his fear when he had always been so self-assured, logical, and brave cast some doubt in my mind. What would happen if he didn't get better?

We got in the car and drove in silence to the hospital. The three of us, together, was the best defense against the fear we all felt. We walked the wide, long hallways of the hospital's first floor, past the gift shop with the pink and blue "Congratulations on Your Baby" balloons, past the coffee shop with nurses taking their breaks.

We walked past the hallway to the cafeteria with its musty smells of old food and burnt coffee. And finally, we made it to the elevator. I wanted to prepare the kids for the hospital room and its grey walls—the IV drip and loud beeping of all the monitors. As we walked by other patients' rooms, I saw them peer in with wide eyes.

I took the lead, walking fast to his room. Inside, my mother and sister were helping him into a wheelchair. He was already dressed in his clothes, the IV removed, the monitors turned off. I exhaled, not realizing I'd been holding my breath for the walk.

"You're all here," he said jovially. He reached up for hugs and I felt a huge relief. He was thinner, yes. Quieter, sure. But he was still so much himself.

"Let's bust me out of here."

We went to his favorite Chinese restaurant— a Szechwan place just five minutes down the road from my childhood home. It was a request he'd made as soon as he knew he was getting out of the hospital. They were releasing him because there was nothing more that could be done. They sent him home to be comfortable in his own surroundings. We sat at a long table in the center of the small room. Steam from the kitchen poured out into the dining area and felt warm and familiar. We held our oversized menus up close to our faces and read the small print, ordered by number, and waited for our food. Nobody mentioned the hospital or cancer or living or dying, and for that one hour, everything seemed okay.

We all drove back to my parent's house after the meal, and everything took a more serious turn. Logistics needed to be solved; we hired a nurse for 24-hour care. We had to go through the mail that had been neglected for the past week. Each one of us took a task, organizing, cleaning, putting things in convenient locations to make his life just a little easier.

"Julie," my dad called out while I was gathering laundry.

"Yeah Papa?"

"Will you come to my office with me?"

I made my way down the stairs to his home office. He looked calm in the big, wood paneled room, surrounded by his papers, his books and vintage calculators. He sat in an old leather chair and called me over to his desk.

"I want to show you where the money is," he said. "I want someone to know about all the accounts and how everything is set up."

"Papa" I started, "Why?"

"Julie," he waved a hand at me. "Just listen."

I took notes. He had watched every penny he had all his life and kept meticulous records that he now shared. He held a shaking finger over each ledger line and explained what went where and how much, just in case he wasn't there to make sure it happened. He had charities picked out. He'd always been generous with non-profit work and good causes.

Now, he listed the Pancreatic Cancer Action Network organization as a recipient of a good sum of money. He wanted to do whatever he could for others, even if he wouldn't directly benefit. I wanted him to tell me that he'd be alive for another 20 years, that he was healthy and happy, and going to fight his way through this. He never said that and deep inside I knew he was right. I was over every day, I made my mom shopping lists with the ingredients she needed to get from the store. I brought over honey and celery and prayed that these purifying foods could keep the cancer at bay. But my dad didn't want to talk about his special diet or if he was hungry or if the pain was getting worse or better. No, he wanted to talk about running. He asked every day how my training was going and how many miles I was doing that week. I'd sit by his side while he laid in bed and tell him about the pace I would need to hit to make it to Boston.

My running shoes had a permanent spot on the porch that led to my father's bedroom. Ever since he was released from the hospital, I wasn't running my normal beach runs, I was doing every mile from that doorstep. I'd breeze into my parent's home, stop and chat and tell my father my proposed mileage for the day. Inside the house, I kept everything light and cheery. Each day, I told my dad, was better than the last. My running was going great, and he was looking better and stronger. Every day, I told him to get ready for Sacramento—we were coming to take over that race and the city.

I arrived on a chilly day to the sound of my mom and dad having some harsh words. He was yelling, exacerbated.

"He's out of control," she said to me as I walked in holding a bushel of celery hearts.

"What is going on?" I said. "Why is he yelling?"

My dad was out of bed, sitting at the kitchen table, looking at a piece of paper. His sweatpants hung off his body, his hands looked like bones.

"Papa. What are you doing? Are you feeling OK?"

"Yes! Why is everyone always asking that? Won't you all just leave me alone and let me make this call?"

"What are you talking about?"

"He got a bill from the dentist," my mom said and threw her hands in the air. "He can't stop talking about it."

"I'm calling the lawyer."

"What? Why, Papa? What would the lawyer have to do with the dentist?"

"He's just being ridiculous," my mom exclaimed.

"I am not," he roared.

"Can you just please tell me what is going on," I said.

"The dentist screwed up my teeth."

"He didn't replace the ones he said they would," my mom said.

"They made a mess."

"So why can't you call them and have them fix it?"

"Trust that so-called dentist again?" He tossed the bill in my direction. "Never."

I picked up the piece of paper off the floor.

"They have the nerve to bill me?" he said. "I'm going to sue his ass."

"For what?" I said.

I could feel heat rising to my face. Mom was right, he was being ridiculous, and totally incorrigible. He didn't seem to understand how inconsequential a dentist's bill was at this moment.

"Papa," I said sweetly.

"No, no Julie. I am not going to calm down or get back in bed or do anything until I call my damn lawyer."

"Jesus, Papa. You sound like a child."

"You don't understand."

I'd heard enough.

"No, you don't understand," I said, my voice raised. "You think this is a joke? Or a game? We're all so worried about you and you want to sue your dentist?"

I slammed the celery down on the counter. My mother looked shocked. I needed to get out of there. I sat down on the step and pulled on one of my running shoes. I'd been doing this same thing for the past week, sitting down on this exact step, and lacing up my shoes before a run. I would usually wait until mile 2, far away from the house, to let any tears I needed to cry come out. But I couldn't help it right then. As I tied my shoes up, I sobbed. I was so mad at him. How could he be so stubborn? But I was more upset at myself. How could I let more negativity into that house? How could I be upset with him?

I'd plotted out a tough four-mile loop from their house. I couldn't see well, my eyes were filled with tears and smeared with mascara, but I stomped ahead anyway. There were hills, so many rolling hills, on the streets around my parent's place in West L.A. I climbed them and rode them down, letting my quads feel the burn and letting myself cry out, "Why?"

Why would my father have to get this diagnosis? Why would it have to happen after we finally had something to share— during a time in my life where I finally felt close to him; like I finally had his approval and love? Why wouldn't my family see the hope I saw? Why was he worrying about his teeth? And why wouldn't I just let him sue the damn dentist?

I also thought of my life right now. Since his diagnosis, I'd been giving myself reasons to pour another glass of wine. I kept dating men that didn't suit me and seemed to repel the nice guys in my life. Even with all the positive changes I'd made, thanks in large part to running, I still needed my father. I wasn't done reconstructing my life. I wanted him around to see the finished product. He needed to wait. I needed him to hold on.

I tackled those hills as though his life depended on it. I ran with determination and sadness. My feet pounded, and my chest felt like it was going to explode. When I felt like I couldn't run another step, I went faster. Running was the only pain I wanted to feel.

It was getting dark by the time I got back to the porch step.

I could see the light on in my father's room. I thought back to nights he would spend in the garage studio, hearing him pounding on the drums and laughing with his brother. I wished he would bring his trumpet out to the porch and sit next to me and play. My legs trembled. God, I thought, this was fucking hard. I wiped the sweat from my forehead and dug my fists into my eyes. I willed myself to stop crying and wiped the mascara from my cheeks. I held my head in my hands for just a second more, and then got up, gathering all the strength I could to walk back through the door and be happy and positive once again.

Inside, he was asleep. I turned off his lamp and tiptoed out of his room. In the kitchen, my mom was dicing celery. Her face was red and I could tell she'd been crying too. I kissed her and said I was heading home for the night. I told her I was sorry. I didn't mean to upset him.

"We're all human, Julie," she said. We were all frustrated. And scared. She hugged me hard.

The call came two weeks later, in the morning.

"Julie," my mom said, "Papa died."

Just fourteen days earlier, we had been yelling at each other about the dentist. Just the night before, he'd asked me about the time of our departing flight to Sacramento.

"No," I said.

"Yes, really, Julie."

I drove, I guess, because somehow, I made it to my mom's side within ten minutes of the call.

"What happened?" I asked her.

"I was out, just for a second," she cried. The nurse had been out as well, just for a moment. He was alone for not even 10 minutes, and he just couldn't hang on anymore. I remember reading about how someone with a fatal illness will wait until they are alone to let go. He'd been struggling with the illness and his pain for so long, and I had been holding onto any hope I could. But he needed to let himself—and all of us—go. The white van arrived shortly after I got there. They loaded his body onto a stretcher and I took his hand. He was covered with a sheet, his face covered as well.

"Papa," I whispered. "Everything is going to be ok. Don't worry, you're just going on a trip." I felt he was scared and didn't know where they were taking him. I needed to hold his hand. Almost like he was a little kid. I just didn't want him to worry or be afraid.

I thought he looked scared and lost, being rolled out of his house by strangers. I held his hand until they were ready to close the van doors.

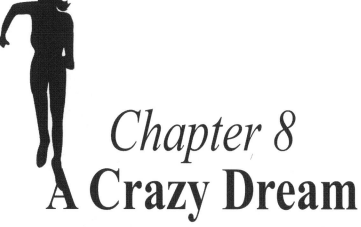

Chapter 8
A Crazy Dream

The marathon was just 10 days away.

The date stirred around in my mind with all the grief and anger, and I couldn't believe I even had to think about running. He was supposed to go with me—to see me finish and reach my ultimate goal. It had been my dad who planted the idea of a BQ in my head, who made me keep fighting for it, and now he was gone. What was the point?

My family hosted a celebration of life in his honor. It was at the family home. The light-filled living room seemed dim. But my mother, light on her feet, seemed to coast from room to room making sure everyone had enough to drink and eat. Playing hostess, keeping herself busy. I appreciated her so much for holding us all in a warm, glowing embrace during the hardest time of her life. We mourned, but we also wanted to give everyone close to Papa a place to rejoice over the full life he led. We wanted music and memories, and conversation that would make him happy.

I got drunk. Wasted, actually. I gave a speech that I don't remember.

David came just before the speech. I took him around, introducing him to my kids, my mom, my ex-husband. We were all there for Papa and I wished so much that David could've met him. I wondered why I never had him over. I also wondered what my dad would've thought about this man I was spending more and more time with. He wasn't anything like Frank, that's for sure. Of course, I knew my father would like him. His drive and his quiet humor, his willingness to help others, his ability to talk to just about anyone and make a connection. My father valued these things. And David was gentle and sweet. I looked at him and put down the glass of wine I'd been clutching. I tried to steady myself and my eyes.

"Want to get some air?" He suggested.

"Sure," I said. Jessie was there, and she needed a walk.

I followed him out the front door. The air felt amazing. It was clear and cool and the sky above was a deep turquoise.

"That was a beautiful speech, Julie."

I laughed. "I don't even know what I said."

"It really captured how great a person your dad was," he said.

For once, we weren't talking about running. We strolled down the sidewalk, along the green lawns and oversized palm trees. We didn't speak for a little while. I felt so close to him. Everything about the moment was perfect.

I stopped. He stopped just ahead of me. I took a few steps closer to him, put my hands on his chest, and we kissed.

###

Race day arrived. I made the voyage to Sacramento and prepared myself to run. This would be the race, I decided. Everyone on the bus was chatting on the way to the start line and there was nervous energy all around. I sat in the back of the bus, quiet for once, saving my energy for the miles ahead. I had one job to do and dammit, I was going to do it. I stopped asking myself why I was running a race so soon after my father died because I knew this was what he would've wanted me to do. I would run the race for him, and I would do it beautifully, too.

The fog of grief cast a shadow around me, but race morning, December 5, 2010, seemed to brighten everything. I actually slept eight hours the night before the marathon, which is unheard of for me. The stars were aligning. The sun shined, the breeze was mellow, and the temperature was just a little chilly—crisp and perfect for a PR.

I ran. I focused every ounce of my energy on putting one foot in front of the other. This time, there were no bold pre-race predictions, no hugs, no thoughts other than the finish. I felt weightless, like I was floating through one mile and then the next. I'd already run 18 marathons and I never felt like this.

When I started out, I clung to the 3:50 pace group and didn't let them out of my sight. I stayed there, matching the pacers stride for stride until both leaders started to struggle.

"Hey," I said. "Are you guys OK?"

"Oh yeah," one said. "You know, I'll probably get a second wind in the next mile."

"I don't know what's going on with me," the other said.

I felt for them. I knew firsthand that the marathon, no matter how prepared you make yourself, can kick your ass. The one who wasn't as optimistic looked pale.

"Do you want me to carry the sign?" I said. Why not? "I'm pretty sure I'm going to run a 3:47."

I wasn't sure where that number came from. That's just

what I thought I would run at that moment.

"No, no," he said. "You're not allowed."

Mile 15 came. The pacers were still struggling, and I couldn't use my energy to worry any longer. Besides, my plan was to start accelerating and take about 30 seconds off my pace per mile. I started to push.

Nothing felt hard. My breathing stayed relaxed, my legs turned over without effort. A light wind caressed my shoulders, as if I was being gently pushed along. Dad, I thought. It pushed me through the next 10 miles. I didn't hit a wall, or feel any pain. I just coasted along, running in a perfect rhythm until I hit the line in 3:47.19—the exact time I predicted.

I pointed skyward as I crossed the finish line, and then dropped to the ground and kissed the earth. I wished that I could have called my dad, I wished that I could have seen and heard him in the crowd, shouting encouragement, but I knew that he was there. I am convinced that we ran my Boston Marathon qualifier— the biggest race of my life, to that point-- together.

I rode that high all the way back to L.A.

My first phone call after the race, the phone call that had always been to my dad, was to David. I knew he would understand just how much this time meant and would be there for me when

I returned. He was thrilled for me and he let me squeal over the phone.

Boston had been on my mind for so long. Because I'd qualified in December 2010—long after the 2011 edition of the race was filled—my qualifying time was for 2012. That seemed too long to wait.

I realized now that I wanted my running to be bigger than me. I felt the hand of Papa again. I'd learned the lessons of charity from him; I'd sat with him in his final weeks as he allocated his money to the causes that he cared about. The Boston Marathon had a rich history of charity runners, and I figured I now had a good reason to try and run to raise money for a good cause.

I applied to Dana Farber, the cancer center in Boston that sponsors marathon racers every year and told them my story. They accepted my application and I was ecstatic. I started training for Boston in April.

Training continued, life continued. That period of time after the loss of a loved one is a haze. Your senses are dulled, you hardly notice you're living. There is the dull ache every day that, whether you realize it or not, slows you down, eats at your core. I kept myself busy pace leading for the L.A. Road Runners, and waited for time to help heal, as everyone said it would.

Running felt like an old friend, there for me whenever I needed it. And every time I ran, I felt like a part of my dad continued to live. I'd talk to him during my training, asking him to help me through Boston, as I felt he had when I qualified; telling him that marathon number 20 was also for him, just as all the others had been.

This time, Maurice Weiss made his presence known in a different way: We raised $10,000 for the race, much of it from the Weiss family foundation. But my dad apparently wasn't inclined to send any breezes my way during the race. Boston is one of the toughest courses I've ever run. Everyone told me to prepare for Heartbreak Hill, but to me, every single incline felt like Heartbreak. I squeaked through just under 4:00. The need to do more came back, stronger than before.

I leaned on David, my coach and my friend. Our relationship grew day after day. He didn't push me or repeatedly demand my love. He was just there for me and I began to develop this deep appreciation for our friendship. And though the haze of grief blurs so much, it also sharpens what is most important. I was no longer reaching for the thrill of a tumultuous relationship. Instead, I started to see who really mattered in my life. My dad had mattered. And now, David really mattered. I couldn't live without him.

I saw in him a beauty I hadn't seen before. I'd been so wrapped up in wanting a tough guy with a tattoo that I was blinded to the attraction I felt for him.

As it grew, we started doing more non-running things together. Going out to dinner, and movies, and events. I invited him to attend a gala that the Pancreatic Cancer Action Network was hosting. This was a cause that had meant much to my father in his last few weeks; and I wanted to support it in any way I could.

The gala was incredible, held at the Beverly Wilshire Hotel in Beverly Hills. Everyone was in their finest clothing, dancing and chatting in the dim evening light. It felt overwhelming, to be in a place where so many people were working to raise money for the same cause--something that had directly affected me and my family.

I sat at our large, round table and stared down at my plate.

"Are you OK?" David asked.

"I am," I said. "I'm just... This whole event feels like I'm meant to be here for some reason, and I'm just not sure why yet."

The band played a slow melody through dinner. I'd hardly eaten and waited in anticipation for a sign I felt was coming. Coffee cups were placed in front of us and servers walked around with regular and decaf carafes. Cake came out on large platters.

Then, the clanking of silverware and mugs softened, and a woman walked up in front of the musicians and took the mic in her hand.

"I hope you're enjoying this party," she said. "It's a wonderful night, and it's important to remember, as we have a good time, why we're all here. We all have something in common--someone we love was impacted by pancreatic cancer."

David grabbed my hand under the table and squeezed.

"There is not much that we can do for this terrible form of cancer," she continued. "We've lost people or have seen our husbands, wives, daughters, sons, mothers, or fathers struggle through the pain. We are powerless to the disease in many ways, but we can take action. And we can do that through research and studies. That's why I am so happy to announce that tonight alone we've raised one million dollars for this cause."

The room erupted in applause. This was an incredible feat. A million dollars in one night.

We left shortly after. I couldn't speak on the drive home. David asked me again if I was OK, and I couldn't explain it to him. I was actually invigorated by the incredible efforts made at the event. And I was awestruck, wanting so badly to contribute in a meaningful way, but not quite sure how to do so. I jumped out of bed the next morning. I had an idea. A crazy, half-baked idea.

What if I were to do something big--really big? Not just one race for money. But 52 races. In 52 weeks. One race per week for a year. I thought about the gala and the funds they raised in just one night. How much could I raise in one year? Wouldn't people be inclined to follow my journey knowing it was for a good cause?

This is it, I thought. I started dancing in my kitchen. A song from the musical "Wicked" popped into my head: "Defying Gravity." I belted it out. My daughter walked into the room and saw me swaying, singing. "Something has changed within me…something is not the same."

"Whoa," she said. "Mother, what is happening here?"

"I had an idea," I told her, still dancing. "I'm so inspired."

I told her what I had planned: 52 marathons in 52 weeks. The more I said it, the more my excitement grew.

"I have so many questions," she said.

"No time for that right now!" I kept singing.

She took out her phone and started filming me. I knew she thought I was nuts, up to another ridiculous running plan. I could see the sly smirk written across her face. She'd grown to be the snarky one in the family. In just a few months, she'd be traveling to Paris for a semester abroad and an adventure of her own. What a perfect intersection in our lives. While she was quiet and subdued much of the time, I could feel her radiating happiness and anticipation. We'd both be exploring a whole new chapter in our lives at the same time. I called David.

"Hey," he answered.

"Hey, I have this half-baked idea."

"Oh yeah?"

"Do you think I can do 52 marathons in 52 weeks?"

He paused. I imagined him on the other end of the line, thinking, calculating, smirking.

"Well, sure," he said finally.

He warned me that I would need to slow down. It wasn't the first time I'd heard him say that. I assured him I would. I told him I would need his help, and he promised he would do whatever it took to get me to the finish of all 52 marathons.

I didn't know it then, but David cemented this idea into reality immediately. He started calling his friends all around L.A. He called people he trained, other coaches, leaders of run clubs and he told them that I was going to do something unbelievable. At this point, and as far as he could discover, very few runners anywhere had done what I proposed to do. His excitement became contagious. Soon, I was getting texts of encouragement. In our circle, there was nothing but positivity. But as soon as he put the word out and it spread, I thought, "shit, I've really got to do this."

That's how David is. His love and excitement for other people, for the sport and the good it can do makes him giddy. I called him again after the rush of greetings came in and asked him how many people he told.

"Just a few."

I was so thankful for a partner in this adventure. I couldn't express it to him at that moment—I was in awe of how generous he was with his time and knowledge.

"Oh, David," I said. "You just signed up to get me through all these races."

Finally, my excitement calmed enough to sit down. It must've been 8 p.m. and with a glass of wine in hand, I grabbed my laptop and settled into a soft couch in my living room. I went to marathonguide.com. The site looks as though it comes from the 1990s. The text is small, the colors faded, and yet it is the best place to find an extraordinary number of marathons, all over the world.

I opened my Outlook calendar. And I started out with the easy ones: anything in Hawaii. I wanted to get back to my running roots as many times as I could. I chose races on my bucket list: New York, Boston, of course. Then, what else? Any race downhill. And there were some that I had never heard of, small races in remote towns--but they happened to fall on open weekends, so they made the list. One weekend, the only race that was scheduled was the Leadville Marathon in Colorado. Rocky Mountains, here I come! And then I chose the Tahoe Triple—three full marathons, in three consecutive days, around the lake, at altitude. Sign me up. Why not? It was easy to choose, based on runner's reviews and my level of excitement. Around 11 p.m., I was done. I shared my calendar with David and wondered about my next steps.

Money, of course, was my first concern. Marathons are expensive pursuits and my goal was to raise funds without going broke in the process. I knew I would need to keep my 9 to 5 as a bookkeeper for Chase Centers Management, a commercial real estate office in Brentwood, just six miles from my home. A gem of a job I couldn't afford to lose, but even my salary wouldn't allow me to register for and travel to all the races I had picked out. I would need some time off, too. I figured I could try to contain some of the trips to weekends, but knew I'd need to take a few Fridays and Mondays. The thought of bringing this up to my boss Rod Chase mortified me.

Rod, the owner of the firm, had already been very supportive of my running (he'd donated a significant amount to my fundraising efforts in Boston). But I was not the type of person to take a lot of personal time, and this would likely use all of my vacation days. I broke into a cold sweat just thinking about it.   But really, how would I swing this financially? I knew if I had the right charity backing me, they might be able to provide some initial funds out of the gate. I figured if I brought funds in, I would be able to justify them spending money on me. I contacted the Pancreatic Cancer Action Network and asked them what I needed to do. I would have to pitch my idea to some of the leaders there. I remembered back to the time I spoke at the public forum about the L.A. Marathon course. I reminded myself that, when I have a cause I believe in, my voice could be strong and convincing. I was amped about this and eager to get going. I reached out to the unofficial Mayor of Running, Bart Yasso—then *Runner's World* magazine's Chief Running Officer, and a beloved figure throughout the sport.

My first question, of course, was, can I do this? Bart, in his infinite wisdom and kindness assured me I could. I figured he must hear a lot of harebrained ideas from runners all over the world, but he knew my story. When I told him about my goal to run 52 marathons in 52 weeks, he said he believed in me and my cause. And he gave me the best piece of advice.

"Start with a bang," he said. "You need a great marathon

to kick this off."

"I thought maybe Boston." I said. "Since that is the mecca."

"Maybe," he said. "I bet you'll know the right race and the right time soon enough."

My head spun. When should I start and when should I tell Rod, my boss? It was clear now that I would need Fridays off, sometimes Mondays, too. He knew me well enough that I could do all my work, no problem. Yet I still feared that conversation and I knew I would need a concrete plan before waltzing into his office and requesting three and four-day weekends for a year. Was I crazy? These thoughts kept me up at night.

Sleeping was never my forte, but now I counted sleepless night after sleepless night. David told me that was no good for the toll my body was going to take. A friend offered meditation tips. And so, there I was, in my small apartment with Jessie by my side, up at 3 a.m. counting to 10, and then back down again. Over and over. It'd only been a matter of days, but already obstacles abounded. A presentation in two days, a hard talk with my boss, and a start date to be decided upon. The uncertainty of the year ahead weighed on me.

And still, David couldn't stop talking about it. Not just to me, but to anyone who would listen. It was cute at first, but now I felt unsure of myself and his constant planning in the abstract left my heart pounding. With little sleep and a pile of stress mounting, I wanted to scream, "cut it out!"

He often came over in the evenings to my apartment. After he was done with work and his track club, and I was done with work, we'd relax on the couch in my shady apartment building. I watched out the window of the second story as he hopped up on the curb. His lanky arms swayed by his side and I could see him smiling, even with the large palm trees blocking most of him. He had good news, I knew it from his stride.

"Julie," he called, nearly singing. He was not even in the door yet.

Jessie ran over to his feet. He crouched down and greeted her.

"You're in a good mood," I said.

"Well," he said. Then he took a deep breath. "Guess who was at the track tonight?"

"Who?"

"It was Gwendolen Twist," he said. "My producer friend. The one who made *Spirit of the Marathon*."

"Oh fun." I figured this accounted for his good mood. David loves that movie, and I do too, of course. The film is like a metaphor for both of our lives—for any marathoner's life, really. It captures what's so amazing about the distance, and Olympic Marathon runner Deena Kastor, who is a total badass, is in it.

"What did she have to say?"

"Well, I told her about the 52."

"Oh, David," I groaned. "You did not."

This was especially embarrassing. Gwendolen Twist, this legendary producer who was fast, like really fast, who-could-qualify-for-Boston-in-her-sleep fast. And David is telling her about my story that hadn't even begun.

"No, no," he said. He put both hands up with a big grin across his face. "Listen to this. They're making another *Spirit of the Marathon*. It's *Spirit of the Marathon II.*"

"Original name."

"I know, I know. But listen, Julie, I told her about the 52 and she wants to interview you."

"What? Why?"

"Because she thought, maybe, no promises, of course, but maybe you might be a good subject in the movie."

"David, shut up."

David coached her for years. I figured she might've said that as a courtesy, but David was insistent.

"I gave her your number and e-mail," he said. "So, I just wanted to let you know in case she calls."

"Oh boy, okay. That sounds…amazing. Thank you, David."

Even if I did have my doubts, I couldn't tell him. He seemed so sure. We ordered in. Italian food from down the street. I devoured pasta with tomato sauce and David picked at his green salad with chicken. Jessie snuggled in between us while we talked. He caught up on my training, asked about my sleep. He just would never get the sleep problems—he was born with a secret talent allowing him to fall asleep just about anywhere, anytime. And then, my phone lit up.

"Oh," I said.

"What is it?" David asked.

"It's Gwendolen, she just texted me. She wants to meet."

"Oh good!"

"At the Loews Hotel on Ocean Boulevard this coming Friday." Two days away. "David, this is nuts. She says she wants to talk about the movie."

"Yup! That's what I said!"

"But I didn't believe you. I thought you were full of it."

We couldn't stop laughing.

"Julie," he said finally. "I don't know why you are not believing in all of this. This mission is important. It's impossible for most people. But you—I know you can do it. That's why I keep telling anyone who will listen."

I couldn't imagine being in a film about running. In *Spirit of the Marathon*, no less. The marathon built me into a woman who felt unstoppable—into someone who wanted to try the impossible.

"Okay," I nodded my head, taking it all in. "Let me respond. Help me respond."

Together, we drafted a text back confirming the meeting. We would meet in the cocktail lounge in the lobby. She said it would be a casual thing, no pressure. I felt the pressure. David put on a pot for tea.

"Let's try chamomile," he said. "You need to sleep."

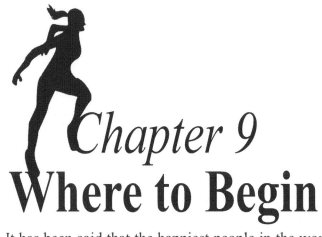

Chapter 9
Where to Begin

It has been said that the happiest people in the world have a goal.

David coached me while he drove through L.A. traffic in his beat-up Lexus. "Take 405," I said, pointing to the exit ramp. He passed it.

"This way will be faster."

The car lurched to a halt at a red light. I stared straight ahead, then into the side mirror. Was my hair tame? My lipstick on right?

David rolled down the window.

"It doesn't matter if you actually achieve that goal, but it does matter that you're going for it. You have an awesome cause you are working for, Julie. And you've got this."

We drove forward, toward the headquarters of the Pancreatic Cancer Action Network. David agreed to take me and my mom, and we were thankful for his support, but he was also driving me crazy with his positive affirmations. My anxiety level felt uncontrollable. My hands tingled, my palms were wet with sweat. I kept rubbing them on my thighs, on the black pencil skirt I'd bought just for this occasion. I needed them to agree to my terms of giving them the money and them basically reimbursing me for travel. I could feel my underarms getting hotter and I prayed I wouldn't sweat through my blouse. And David, he wouldn't go the way I wanted him to, and I got annoyed and he just kept talking.

"Julie, don't worry," he said. "Stop yelling at me. We will make it there right on time."

I should be grateful, I reminded myself. He is such a good person. But what I needed at that moment was a second of silence. I was about to go into a corporate building and basically put my hand out. I closed my eyes, "You've got this, you've got this, you've got this."

The night before, I had created color-coded Excel spreadsheets showing how I thought all the donations would come in and the sponsors we could get. David was right, there was interest and this mission could catch people's attention.

Making the spreadsheets, I felt at home. Uniting my two passions—raising money for the illness that took my father's life and running—seemed like my purpose in life at that moment. I gathered my running credentials: 12 marathons in 12 months, 20 marathons total, a pace leader for the largest running group in LA. Plus, I was a mom, a full-time accountant, and I was pretty good at talking to the media. "Make me the face of the Pancreatic Cancer Action Network!" That was my pitch. Put me out there, I'll run a marathon a week for a year (somehow), get a lot of attention and together we can raise a crapload of money.

Purple is the color for pancreatic cancer awareness, and I wore a purple shirt, a wristband, and purple nail polish. It was my favorite color and there wasn't a day I didn't wear it. I combed through my hair, wiped my hands down my tights again. David was still talking.

"This is a dream," I could hear him saying as I tried to practice the breathing techniques I'd mastered. "And this is your chance to make it a reality." No pressure, I thought.

We pulled into the parking lot. We were early by 15 minutes, but I needed to get out of the car.

"Okay, bye," I almost sprinted away, my heels clicked

through the parking lot. My mom trailed behind me. As I waltzed through the front doors of the building, I breathed deep and hard.

Three people met with me. I don't even remember if I made it through the whole presentation. But I remember the handshakes and hugs after. The Pancreatic Cancer Action Network would be my allies through this journey. They would sponsor some of my mission. I asked for one more thing: a running shirt to represent them at every race. The board members laughed. They could do that.

One down, one to go. At work, I stared at photo stills from *Spirit of the Marathon*. That evening, I would meet with the director and would plead my case. But this was more than a presentation about my cause. This was an audition. So many variables at play: would I fit the mold they were casting for? Was I fit enough, pretty enough, interesting enough?

I practiced faces in the mirror. My smile, my laugh. Would these expressions translate on camera? This was L.A. after all, and even if it was a movie about runners, I figured they would want people who were easy to look at. I was thankful for all the good running had done to my body, though I knew I wasn't what a traditional runner looked like. David was shaped like a runner: long, lean limbs and gaunt cheekbones. I had hips, a butt, sculpted legs, and curves. Yes, I had enhanced my breasts after my daughter was born, and I loved my implants. They made me feel womanly, and I didn't care if people judged me for paying attention to my appearance, I did what made me feel good. And what would make me feel good now would be to carry the banner of pancreatic cancer awareness to thousands of my fellow runners who would watch this movie. I thought I could fill that role well, but what would the producers think?

I drove myself. David would wait at the apartment with Jessie and I would let them know how it went. "We will either meet for a celebratory meal, or we will drink tea on the couch to mourn," I told him and kissed him goodbye.

"You're going to be great!" He assured me.

At the hotel, I headed to the cocktail bar where we were supposed to meet. When I arrived, both Jon Dunham the director and Gwendolen Twist were already there, on a couch in the lobby by the cocktail bar. They both had pinkish martinis.

"I'll have what they're having," I said to the waitress.

I sat at a table, took a sip, and instantly felt my shoulders relax. It was cold, and flowery, and refreshing. Ever since David and I started dating, I'd been drinking more tea than wine. The last glass I poured was while I mapped out my marathon year, and

I hardly touched it since I was so preoccupied with the dates and logistics. This drink, being just the right amount of sweet, tasted amazing.

I could feel the alcohol rushing to my head. I knew my cheeks were red. Even in my drinking days, hard liquor went straight through me. *You are not drunk.* I yelled inside my head. *You're buzzed. Buzzed is okay.*

"Let me buy you another," Gwendolen said when I finished my first drink. She smiled warmly, her dirty blonde hair whipping around her face as she got the attention of our server. I told myself I would just sip it. Refusing would be rude.

"How are you?" I said again. *A double greeting? She's going to think you're some airhead with nothing to say!*

"I'm great. I am just so happy we're getting to talk. David said so many great things about you."

"Oh, that's David for you," I said. "He probably made me sound much better than I actually am." I took another sip. *Why? Why am I drinking more? Am I slurring my words?*

I tried to get a hold of myself and my nerves. I spoke slowly, enunciating dramatically and asked Gwendolen about her running while I gulped ice water.

I talked about the plan, the mission, and let loose in a way

I hadn't with anyone before. My honesty felt shocking. I told them about my doubts and the anxiety. I told them about the sleepless nights and how meditating felt like bullshit at the current moment.

I went on and on about Jessie, that fluff ball, who was my first and greatest running partner. And I confessed that even with a plan in place, I had no idea where to begin. What race would be worthy of this mission, what could possibly kick this off?

They nodded and asked questions.

"You have kids?"

"Yes! Two. Samantha and Frankie. Samantha is going to be in Paris this semester. Frankie thinks I'm a total nut for doing the 52, but they always think I'm a little off."

"What do you do for work?"

"I'm a bookkeeper. A master of Excel. It's my not-so-secret superpower."

I told them about running in Hawaii when I was depressed and overweight. I told them about my life with the L.A. Road Runners, how I ran 12 marathons in 12 months, and how I never stopped until I qualified for Boston. And then I told them about Papa.

"He was my biggest support, my unofficial coach," I told them. "And I just woke up one morning after he died and realized

I had to do something bigger than myself. To honor him. And he was so pleased with my running, I just… I wanted to run for him."

I got emotional about my father and Gwendolen took my hand while I wiped tears away. With my second drink finished, and the night growing long, we all said goodbye. Gwendolen said she would call me in a day or so to let me know. They told me that they planned to start shooting the film right away, that the race was less than two months away, in March, in Rome.

"Rome? Now, that would be a helluva way to start this journey," I said and laughed. They laughed too and said goodbye. I climbed into my car, kicked off my heels. I replayed the last sentence I said over and over. *Was I being too presumptuous? Did they think I thought that I already had the role?*

I hit rewind on the night. I had just invited myself to their movie, I talked too much, was probably too loud and possibly drunk. I laughed. I laughed a lot. This was not the collected version of myself I'd practiced in the bathroom mirror. These people were looking for refined runners, people who could live up to Deena Kastor's eloquent ruminations on the marathon in the first movie. *You blew it*! My inner critic said. I put my head on the steering wheel. *You had to have that second drink?* I took out my cell and called David.

"I think I need a ride home."

"How did it go?" David asked.

"You won't be seeing me in any movie any time soon."

####

Helicopters whirred overhead. A crane, 30-feet high, loomed above us, rising out from a distant street, over the Vatican, aimed at the crowd of people on the street. The start line of the 2012 Maratona di Roma. The staging area of any marathon is one of the most emotional, incredible places—each start comes with its own fears, challenges, waves of excitement. But this wasn't just any marathon. This was a marathon in the ancient city; and the marathon that was being used as the setting for a major motion picture on the sport.

And I was in it! As the pack pressed forward, eager for the start, I thought back on the whirlwind of events since the night I drank and laughed and double-greeted my way out of a role in this movie.

I was wrong.

Two weeks after that night, we got the news that I'd been selected. David and I both shrieked with excitement.

"This is going to kick off the 52!" I exclaimed. "Rome will be number one!"

I couldn't celebrate long because March was around the corner and the planning needed to start. To start, I still needed to talk to my boss, I needed marathons scheduled right after Rome, and I needed races close to home as well. I would need media attention to get the word out, to help the Pancreatic Cancer Action Network, and to help get other potenial sponsors on board. I needed plane tickets, and new shoes, and miles of training. "You're going to be fine," David told me as I paced around the apartment soon after the phone call. He studied the computer, looking for all the races in between Rome and Boston.

I went to work with this big secret bubbling inside me. Each day, I'd look down at my hands while inputting code into spreadsheets and catch a glimpse of my purple nail polish. I would smile. And then I would panic. I needed to walk into Rod's office and ask for permission. I needed him to know that in addition to the time off, I would likely be exhausted for the next year, and I would probably be wearing running shoes to the office.

When I couldn't take it anymore, I walked into Rod's office and sat down. He is a very kind, sweet and generous man, but he also has a business to operate.

"I'm running 52 marathons in 52 weeks in honor of my dad and I'm probably going to need to take a lot of Friday afternoons off, and some Mondays, but not a lot of Mondays, and I will still do all my work," I said.

I handed him my tentative calendar. He considered this rapid-fire information and flipped through the calendar.

"Well," he said.

"Well?"

"I mean, I think you have the vacation time. And I know you're a hard worker." He thought for a moment, rubbing his temple with his pen. "This is a pretty ambitious goal."

He was thinking aloud. Likely calculating the distances, the miles, the air travel.

"You're really going to do this?"

"Yes, I'm raising money," I said.

"Let's see how it goes."

"Okay," I said.

"As long as you think you can still do your job and get your work done," he said, "go for it."

That was it. I felt like with that approval, I was all in.

I invited cameras into my home and they filmed me running along the beach, next to the Santa Monica Pier. I made sure they got good footage of Jessie and showed David trying to torture me with foam rollers. I told them my story, showed them old photos of Papa. The more I talked about my dad, the more I thought about the arc of our relationship. He'd caused me pain, but I did the same to him. Those lost years where I did nothing but disappoint my family remained a great burden on my conscience. Sometimes, I couldn't shake the smell of pot and stale beer from my memories. I was so sorry for all the worrying he and my mom must've experienced. But I tried to remember the good times too. I could hear the drums playing from the garage, still. And I was so grateful that running, in the end, was what mended old wounds. I knew, also, that the old showman would have been delighted to see me co-starring in a big show like this. At the start line, the crowd lurched forward, little by little. We stood in a pack, shoulder to shoulder.

"Can you believe it's about to begin?" David whispered to me and held my hand. Something else happened too before we even started the 52. In a weekend in Chicago, David had proposed. I was so in love with this man, and I immediately accepted. He gave me a beautiful ring that belonged to his mother, and I was happy to show it off in Italy. My family loved David—my daughter especially. He was our rock, our calming presence, and now my sidekick in this crazy adventure.

The start of one marathon is stressful enough. But as we waited those last seconds, I realized that this was the start of something even grander—and scarier! Fifty-two marathons in fifty-two weeks. Was I completely crazy to even attempt this? Just then, the Rome Marathon's theme song, Dean Martin's "That's Amore" blared from the speakers, and David twirled me around, and dipped me back. I squealed, feeling like a teenage girl in love, while runners sidestepped us, and looked on with amusement.

The packed crowd moved slowly toward the start line. Despite how good I felt and how confident I was in my body's ability to take me through 26.2 miles yet again, those same thoughts that everyone has at the beginning of a race lingered. Could I finish? Would I hit a wall? Would something unpredictable happen—a sprained ankle? A flash flood? The sudden need to go to the bathroom? To make matters worse, cameras would capture nearly everything.

We decided to start closer to the back since, as David mercilessly reminded me, we needed to go slow. Around us, the Italian runners wished one another luck. *In bocca al lupo!* They said. (Translation: "into the wolf's mouth," the Italian equivalent of "break a leg.") I heard it so often, I started saying it myself. I shook hands and high fived so many runners as we made our way over the start mat, and then, just like that, our journey to 1,362.4 total miles in 52 weeks was underway.

Holy crap.

I couldn't control my delight. God, it felt good to run. The streets, lined with ancient ruins and beautiful architecture, made my heart swell. I thought of how much my parents would love to be there with me. My dad, maybe playing his trumpet next to some of the bands that lined the course—I could picture him on the street, cheering me on and chatting with the spectators.

I took big leaps over potholes. I danced with runners who held out their hands. It was early in the race and my legs felt good. My adrenaline pumped, hard. This wasn't just 26.2 miles, I kept reminding myself and somehow that made my body want to push harder and faster.

"Julie," I would hear David behind me, diligently keeping a nice, easy pace. "You should slow down a bit."

The course was marked by kilometers, but my trusty watch alerted me to mile marks. The first few flew by.

"Okay! This is a great pace," I kept my voice cheery and light and trucked along with them at a clip that felt painfully slow. With my watch sounding through the miles, I counted 13 beeps and knew the Vatican would be approaching soon.

Ancient churches lined the cobblestone streets as we approached. I could see the history, with the passage of time feeling massive and incomprehensible. Then, around a corner, the Vatican appeared—a small city burning in our eyes. I fell back with my pack and took it in with them.

Just beyond the 14-mile mark, David calmly said my name.

"Honey, my foot felt a little weird on one of those cobble-stones."

"Okay," I said, urging him to explain a little more.

"Well, it makes me think about Abebe Bikila."

"What?"

"The Ethiopian runner who ran barefoot in the 1960 Olympics here. He won."

Leave it David to tell me about history in the middle of a marathon.

"But even wearing shoes, those roads got me," he continued. "And I think my left foot might be sprained. Maybe broken."

"Broken?"

"Yeah," he said. "I mean, it feels better now, on the paved roads."

I felt okay still, for the moment, but I felt so bad for David. I apologized for going out too fast and for speeding up to reach the Vatican.

We forged ahead. I clapped for the bands, checked on David's pain level, sprinted ahead, then turned back. I held out my arms into the shape of airplane wings and swerved through the runners, hoping to give everyone a good laugh. This felt easy and I wondered if the middle of a marathon pack was my place in the world. Each step made me feel stronger, happier, more complete. I thought that maybe every race would be as joyous as this first one. I remembered the heartache of missing BQ's, of running close to four hours but never breaking it. I thought that maybe the pain of 26.2 miles was more mental and that my legs could easily carry me through all 52 without the agony I'd suffered in the past. It was, at the very least, a nice thought to have at the moment.

"C'mon everybody!" I yelled, cheering for anyone who looked like they needed an extra boost.

I approached a diminutive Italian man, who appeared to be in his 60s or 70s, and, towering over him, smiled down.

"Hey! Good job!" I yelled, even though he was right there, the miles behind me clouding some of my judgement. "We've got this!"

He responded in Italian, and I figured he was saying something like "thank you." celebrating, too. We were well past the 20-mile mark, in the homestretch. The energy in those last miles of a marathon is a strange mix. You know you've almost made it, and you're wanting to pick it up, but you're also worn down, dog tired, and your mind and heart and body create some confusion. You might want to go faster and celebrate, but sometimes, you just can't.

Later, I found out that the little old man I'd been hovering over was basically telling me to keep my mouth shut. "Don't talk," he had said to me in Italian. "It will make you tired." He stayed on my heels as we rounded corners and ticked off more kilometers. I still felt strong, amazing actually. And then, by the Trevi Fountain, the finish line appeared. With David and the old man trailing right behind me, I crossed the line, hands up, feeling elated.

David grabbed me for a kiss. The old, Italian man offered me a hug. Even though he had some sage advice for me during the marathon—advice that can essentially be translated to: "shut the hell up!" I think my positivity helped him finish in good spirits. "We've got this!" I said to him. I'm not sure he knew what that meant, nor am I sure myself. But I liked that expression and vowed to use it again and again. I wanted everyone to know that this wasn't a solo adventure. In every race, we're running together. "We've got this," became my new favorite phrase.

We drank champagne from plastic stemware. Boston would be next. Just 51 to go.

Chapter 10
First Steps on a
Long Journey

Sweat dripped down my forehead into my eyes and I hoped
like hell my mascara wouldn't run into my eyes. My watch read 9
a.m. and yet the sun shone above us like high noon. The temperature crept upwards (it was projected to hit a high of 90) and I hid
under the shade of some trees in Hopkinton.

This was Boston in April? It felt more like Palm Springs
in July. Every day leading up to race number two, I checked the
weather, hoping to see a change. Don't get me wrong, I live for sun
and warmth. But for 26.2 miles I would gladly take a typical New
England day in the spring. The marathon gods had other things in

store for the Boston runners and I had a job to do. I tried my best to put the heat out of my mind.

Boarding the bus on the way to the start, I couldn't help but hold my head high. This was the Boston I earned; the culmination of my BQ attempts. I imagined calling my dad to tell him, "Hey Papa, I finally made it," or even him actually here, cheering me on through Heartbreak Hill. I could feel his presence and his blessing. More than anything, I could feel him shining through me as I started chatting with the other runners on the bus.

I turned from one stranger to the next to get the read on the race. One person I met, David Kahn, was a big teddy bear of a man from Birmingham, Alabama with a lively Southern accent. He told me he was running his first marathon for a charity called Team Meb, which focuses on health, education and fitness initiatives around the world. Boston is magical in that way—not only are there so many folks who are fast as hell, there are also runners so dedicated to their cause that they train while raising money to race the Boston marathon and benefit their charity.

David told me his story, and I couldn't help but go on about mine. My voice sounded more like a squeal as I explained that today would be marathon number two. "I'll do 50 more this year," I told him.

In the Athlete's Village, I coasted around from one shady spot to another, looking for my friend, Dino. I knew Dino mostly from our posts back and forth on social media. We shared a connection. His father, too, had died from pancreatic cancer and he now dedicated his running life to the cause, just as I was doing. Athlete's Village is a strange place. Big screen TV's and blaring music created visible waves in the sticky heat. Rows of porta potties were all around me.

I heard someone yell my name and turned around to see Michael Gilman, one of the men in my pace group, waving to me from across the lawn. I loved seeing people who I knew from my small piece of the running world. And I loved meeting people who I only knew through profile pictures and written notes on Messenger. In Boston, everyone comes together—all parts of the running community.

But it was Dino who I needed to find because he was the founder of Project Purple, the biggest running-pancreatic cancer nonprofit in the country. I wanted to share in his cause, and besides, it was his first race and I told him I would run it with him.

I knew I would have to take Boston even slower than Rome. David had of course given me grief about my unrelenting pace down the cobblestone streets of Rome. His "broken" foot ended up being fine. The race timing pod had gotten lodged between his foot and the upper fabric of the shoe, but I still felt guilty for speeding down the road while he hobbled along. This race, I decided, would be different. I would stop worrying about my time so much. A five-hour marathon is a five-hour marathon. I wasn't trying to set any PRs—I had a bigger goal. That's at least what I kept repeating to myself.

In the crowd, a man's face stood out. Dimples and dark hair. Dino's rakish smile, slightly more lifted on the left side, lit up across his face.

"Dino!" I shouted. He waved and started walking toward me, a purple body in a sea of Boston's traditional blue and yellow.

"Julie." He leaned in for a brief hug. We both had sweat pouring from us and the race had not even started. "This is going to be rough, isn't it?"

"We're just gonna take it easy," I said. I tried to sound reassuring.

The day before, when we met in the lobby of my hotel in downtown Boston, we had agreed to run 11-minute miles. Any experienced marathoner would adjust their plan because of the rising heat. I cautioned Dino against going out too fast and thought of my upcoming weeks, the races ahead. I knew I couldn't risk dehydration. Yes, we decided, we would move slower. At a sloth-like pace. "As long as we make it to the finish, we've got this." Dino agreed.

His dad, Giovanni, was a fighter. His first bout with pancreatic cancer was in 2008 and Dino watched as his dad underwent chemotherapy and surgeries. His body grew pale and weak, but the spark in his eye—I imagine the same spark Dino has—remained. Against the odds, the treatments worked. In remission, he could eat again and his skin turned from yellow to a glowing olive. But here's the thing: the rate for pancreatic cancer survival after five years is just nine percent, which according to the National Cancer Institute makes it the most lethal form of the disease. The Verrelli family was cautiously optimistic but knew the time they had together was a gift. In 2010, the cancer returned and this time it was too advanced for treatment.

The helplessness you feel in that moment is so unbearable you just want to scream. When Dino explained it to me, I just wanted to reach out and embrace him. I knew that feeling too well. To hear them get a death sentence, and to have to stand by, hoping for a miracle. It could break you. Or, you could devote your life to ending the disease that took them. That, I reminded myself, was a big part of why I was here in Boston prepared to run 26.2 miles on a sweltering hot day, a week after running another marathon. Dino promised his dad he would never stop fighting. Boston was his first goal. I was so proud to be standing at the start with him.

"This is for Maurice and Giovanni," I said as we cruised through mile one. We were caught up in everything—the energy of Boston, the beauty and tragedy of our own personal battles, and the greater good we hoped we were doing. I saw him look down at his watch as we approached mile two.

"Uh oh."

"What?"

"We're going too fast," he said. We must've been going at a ten-minute clip. "I feel really good," I said. Of course, I felt really good. It was only mile two and the first part of the Boston Marathon course is slightly downhill. "Are we on pace?"

"Nope," he said. I wanted to tell him he was probably psyching himself out, that we should run what feels right. This was Boston after all, the fittest runners took this course on, and I didn't want to be a disgrace to the race. I earned my spot here. Then I remembered it was Dino's first marathon. And it felt like 100 degrees.

"Oh, let's slow down then," I said, probably with too much enthusiasm. "Less than 24 miles to go!""

"Julie, I don't know how you have so much energy."

Neighbors on the course set up water stops. The firemen opened hydrants. Torrents of water appeared like mirages, wavy in the distance, but they were real, and so glorious each time we reached them. I praised people with thanks, chatted with spectators. I high-fived other runners and yelled at nearly every runner that they were amazing. Dino drank with unquenchable thirst. By mile nine, I was still riding a high. Dino had stopped talking.

"You're a rock star! I yelled. "Keep going."

He was tired. He was also grumpy. I replayed the miles before and thought back to the old Italian man who'd basically told me to shut up, that I would make myself tired. He was a grump, too. But he had a point—my positivity and volume level could be, well, annoying. Especially for someone who had to hear it for nine miles.

I stopped my loud cheering and fell into Dino's cadence.

"How are you doing, friend?"

"Fine, tired."

David had packed my fuel belt full of mineral pills and gave me instructions to take them at the first signs of dehydration. I felt in tune with my body and knew that to get through the rest of the race, taking one would help. I looked over at Dino's body. He was hunched over, his dimples flattened out by the look of agony on his face. His purple singlet was drenched, turned to a deep plum. I handed him a mineral pill, explained that severe dehydration could lead to sodium depletion. I thought of the amount of water he'd chugged so far. He took it and looked at me with a grateful smile. Okay, I thought. Maybe I redeemed myself for being so irritating. I handed them out to other struggling runners. No one needed to die today.

"How are we doing Dino?" I yelled. "You're doing amazing."

We slugged along. The sun beat down on us, the water stops continued to be our saving grace. I saved my energy, growing concerned for everyone, including myself, about the Newton Hills. I'd studied the Boston course even before I qualified, and I knew more about the lure of this race than any other event in sports. David and I liked to trade stories of the Boston legends. For me it is Kathrine Switzer, the first woman to run Boston with a bib number. David loved to talk about Alberto Salazar and Dick Beardsley's extraordinary neck-to-neck race now called (thanks to Jon Brant's eponymous book about that epic competition, Duel in the Sun).

We were marathon dorks and we knew it. But on a day like today, it was useful to know the agony that was about to come. Even though Boston is a net downhill course, the ups and downs past mile 18 are treacherous. Here, as Dino and I passed the 16-mile mark, I wanted to prep him for what was about to come. I mustered up the courage to act like David—the fearless pacer. But before I could open my mouth, Dino dropped to a walk.

I stopped, too.

"You go on," he said. "I won't be able to hold a steady pace for the rest of the race."

He reached his arms up and laid his palms flat against the nape of his neck. Around us, most of the runners had slowed to a walk, or at best, to a shuffle. Dino tried to breathe deeply, slowly regaining control of his breath.

"No," I said. This wasn't up for debate, I assured him. I would get him through Heartbreak Hill and then I would break off, if I was still feeling good. I wouldn't take a chance on leaving him before we encountered the hardest part of the course. Heartbreak Hill is filled with stories of people who broke down. The ascent is a steady nearly-half mile climb. While that's tough enough, what makes Heartbreak so feared by runners is that it comes last in the race, between miles 20 and 21, the last of the four Newton Hills. My first time running Boston, I kept wondering which hill was the infamous Heartbreak. They all sucked. The first is around mile 16, a difficult point on the course, where many hit the wall, running out of glycogen for fuel. It was there where John Kelley overtook Ellison Brown, in 1936, patting him on the shoulder. The gesture motivated Brown to rally back, passing the defending champ Kelley, and continue on to win the race. It's said that this broke Kelley's heart, hence the name of the hill. I would have happily told Dino this story, but I suspected he just needed me to be quiet.

We battled through each climb, quads burning on the descents. On the uphills, I closed my eyes. I saw the long hallway in my childhood home. I imagined running my fingers along the plaster on the walls, feeling the rough texture, walking slowly, deliberately, from the living room back to my dad's bedroom. Light poured into the windows, light as bright and suffocating as the sun beaming down on me here in Boston. I shut my eyes tighter and envisioned him in bed, near the end. A big man, despite his wasting body, feet nearly touching the bed frame, a single sheet covering him, and a weak smile greeting me.

Heartbreak Hill was just ahead. I grabbed a 5-hour energy drink and downed it in a single sip. Dino nodded, step after step, and I told him he was close to done, that this was the worst part, that it was very literally a cake walk compared to the miles we just did. We flew up that damn hill, and I zigzagged, arms out like an airplane, as I had in Rome, feeling invincible and strong. The crowd roared. Dino likely rolled his eyes. Any pain I was feeling, I told myself, was nothing compared to what my father went through, and so I channeled his love of life, his great presence, and charged up, breaking that hill like it had broken others.

I knew Dino would finish the last six miles. I needed to be tough now—to set the tone for the rest of the journey. I knew, too, that our plane back to L.A. would leave in just five hours, no time to visit the Cheers bar. So I said good bye to my friend and ran as fast as I could for the finish line. 5:08. My finish time. I threw up my Goddess arms, crossed the line, and searched for David. We wouldn't have a second to spare.

Hotel. Smoothie. Shower. Airport. That's how quickly we moved. It was quite a bit different from the elaborate champagne toast and leisurely recovery in Rome. This, I understood suddenly, would be my new life. On the plane, I took out a foam roller and worked out my legs in the aisle. I went to the galley, got on the floor and moved through a few forward folds and downward dogs. My legs burned. My temperature was still high. I didn't care what the other passengers thought.

I sat back, wishing I could call my dad. I would tell him that I just finished the hottest Boston on record at 89 degrees. I threw one leg across David and the other in the aisle and watched

194 | Julie Weiss

him fall asleep in his seat. We had just started on an incredible journey of love, hope, inspiration and achy legs. Next up, the San Luis Obispo Marathon. I had six days to recover.

Chapter 11
The Colorado River

I sat at work with my feet out of my running shoes, staring at my computer screen. My shirt was wrinkled, and I keep running my palms down the front of it, hoping nobody could notice the deep creases. It hurt to move my arms. In my peripheral view, I caught a co-worker looking at me with concern and hoped she wouldn't get up from her desk and come over. My brain felt fuzzy. The burnt coffee smell that wafted out of the break room turned my stomach. I glared back at the well-meaning coworker. She had stopped asking about the races after Boston. Two races deserved celebration. Five in five weeks—asking gets tiring. I got it.

It was Friday. The past three races had all been in California and staying close to home was a gift. The showers in my own bathroom, the meals I could choose, time on the couch with Jessie.

But the very next day, that would all end. David and I would haul off to Palisade, Colorado for the Grand Valley Marathon, a race I'd never heard of in a place that sounded far, far away to me.

I checked my donations page again. The number was still at a disappointing $50,000. I had promised one million.

Hunger, really more like immediate starvation, struck. I opened my snack drawer and grabbed everything in sight. I slowly unwrapped a protein bar, trying not to make the wrapper crinkle, trying not to spill chocolate down the front of my wrinkled shirt. Eating will take me five minutes, I reasoned, and then it will be 4:49 p.m., near enough to closing. Time to leave.

At home, my suitcase was out and David had already put in some essentials. My Pancreatic Cancer Action Network sports bras and singlet, a few pairs of shorts, socks, water bottles. I stared down at the contents of the suitcase longing for the days when it symbolized a vacation—perhaps to Hawaii.

David buzzed around me, readying my other belongings, visibly more excited than I was about this next marathon. I collapsed on the couch.

He stopped for a moment. "What's wrong?"

"It's the donations," I said. "They're not coming in."

He stopped packing to reflect on this for a moment, in his

calculating, logical way. "Julie, it's only been four marathons. It's so early in the process."

I closed my eyes and waited for him to resume his frantic packing.

"You keep…ugh," I start. "You're flittering around all over."

"I'm packing for you."

"I can pack myself. I have everything all ready."

"Okay, okay."

"Just, let's have an early night," I said. "What time are we leaving for the airport tomorrow?"

"Whenever you want."

It was a Saturday flight, and traffic to LAX is notoriously bad, no matter when you go. I knew David had his training group in the morning, and he would likely have time to kick it off and head back to pick me up. I agreed to be ready and waiting for him. I drifted to sleep easily. Exhaustion was at least allowing me to get to bed on time.

Frustration stirred me out of bed. I woke up late and I woke up angry. What was I angry about? I didn't know. I was mad that I had to get on a plane, annoyed that David wasn't there. This wasn't fair, I know. I told him to go to the training group, and I was the one who signed up for this madness. But logic didn't help me settle down. I stomped through the apartment, gathering my things, glancing out the window and expected David to arrive in his clunky Lexus at any time.

Minutes ticked by. Where was he?

I paced. I checked our tickets, checked the clock on the oven, then looked out the window. I repeated this sequence as the numbers ticked up. "We're going to be late," I grumbled to myself. This was the only plane leaving LAX for Colorado that day, and I needed this marathon to keep the 52 going. Panic set in. I grabbed all the bags. I would be ready when he came. I started hurling them down the stairs.

I couldn't hold back: I chucked one bag after another letting out pathetic little gasps as they thumped down the apartment steps and hit the door to the outside.

"Julie," I heard David call from the bottom.

"Oh, you're finally here."

I started stomping down the steps, kicking a backpack that hadn't reached the bottom. David didn't look for an explanation or try to calm me down. He just picked up the bags and brought them to the back seat of his car.

"You know," I said icily, "it would be easier to load the car if you ever cleaned out your trunk."

Why was I picking on David right now? He looked up at me with a sympathetic smile. "We're going to make it, Julie, I promise."

I was silent on the way to the airport. David whirred down the highway, speeding and swerving around traffic, suddenly realizing just how late we really were. I knew we were going to have to run from our parking lot to the terminal. I didn't know if my body could handle a sprint to the plane. We hit traffic, of course. I logged onto the airport schedule and searched flights that took us anywhere near Grand Junction, Colorado, close to the race start. But those square states are big and vast with lots of miles in between major cities.

"If we don't make this flight, we won't make this race."

I spoke in a strange, calm robotic tone that I never heard myself use before. I was furious, rage boiling inside me. Why couldn't he have just gotten back to the house on time? Why couldn't there be another race in California this weekend? Soon, I was mad at the entire state of Colorado.

We sprinted. We hustled. We made it to the gate just before they shut the cabin doors. The two of us sat through the flight without saying a word.

The upcoming 26.2 would be a true test. I was in no condition to run a marathon—mentally, physically, spiritually. I was a zombie merely dragging myself through the motions. We drove from the airport deeper and deeper into the mountains. Buildings became fewer. The great pines emerged from the earth like towering, green pyramids. I know that some people are called to the mountains the way I am to the ocean. I tried to let the magic of the Rockies calm me, and I called to them internally. But all I felt was an echo of loneliness. God, I was tired.

"What time is the race?"

"He speaks!"

It was the first sentence David uttered from the time we hit the road.

"I know you're beat," he said. "I didn't want to bug you."

How could he be so understanding? Doesn't he understand all this patience and kindness is just going to get me more ticked off?

"It starts at 7:00 a.m. sharp," I said. "I'm going to sleep." I figured I would pass out before this kind, empathetic man said another nice thing and I attacked him for being too good to me. I was a mess, I knew it and he knew it. I figured I would wake up, have a nice, leisurely breakfast, run the race easy and have five done. Five marathons out of 52 would make me feel better, I was sure of it.

We left the hotel to find the start at 6:30 a.m. I had tossed and turned a bit but managed to get a solid four hours of sleep, which was much better than some nights before a race. We twisted down a single-lane road in Grand Junction, a small spot on the map about four hours west of Denver. The tiny downtown looked like a movie set from some old Western. When we approached the start line, no one except a few volunteers were there. I knew the race was small, but I didn't think I'd be the only participant..

"Hi," I approached a man who looked like he was in charge.

"Hey there!" He shook my hand and smiled. "Running behind?"

"What's that?"

"You're a little late," he said with a laugh.

"Late?" David asked.

"What time did it start?" My panic set in. We had just made the flight, we traveled miles to get to this tiny town, and now I was about to mess up this whole weekend because I couldn't read race day information?

"The gun went off at 6:30 a.m. sharp," he said. He checked his watch. "Just about 15 minutes ago…"

"Oh my God. I thought it started at 7 a.m. Can I still run?"

"Well yeah, girl," he said. "You probably won't win, but

you can definitely run."

"I don't have a bib. I don't have anything."

"Don't worry, you go on ahead and I'll get you sorted out."

There was no chip timing in this race; no technology, just a big, glowing red clock. The rest of the race had a 15-minute head start. I figured that I might finish dead freaking last, but that didn't matter. I set out steady and slow. I needed to calm my breath and get my heart rate down after the stress of being late. At least they had let me run!

As I ran down the middle of the road, all alone, I listened to the Colorado River roaring along next to me. Then, in front of me, a lone man waved his arms frantically. He was thin and tall. And he looked kind of like David.

"What are you doing out here?" I ran up to him, panting a bit, surprised to see him out on the course. "How did you even get here?" We were at mile two.

He didn't bother to answer. Instead, he showed me my race bib in his hand and pinned it to my shirt. I wouldn't have been an official finisher without it, ending my streak right then and there. "Oh David." I cried. How could I have been so terrible to him? Who cares if his car is a mess or that he doesn't understand the concept of traffic in L.A. (he is from Ohio after all)?

"Think about it like a training run," he said, always the coach. "It's amazing out here, enjoy it."

I spent the next several miles keeping a steady, easy pace. The air was pine-filled and crisp. I got myself in the moment and focused on my stride and the old fundamentals of running. There was no one out there to cheer, no cameras following me, no running partners to annoy with my constant chatter. Just me and the road, the mountains, and the river.

For the first time in a while, I went easy on myself. A big hill approached, and I decided to walk up. I tried to take a deep breath, but the thinness of the air made me choke a bit. This is okay, I thought. This is how this race is supposed to be and the universe is telling you to slow down. As I continued along, I saw a person ahead of me.

"Hey!" I said, excited to see someone out on the course. "Are you running the marathon?"

"Run-walkin' it," she said and smiled. "Next week, I have an ultra, so I'm just getting some miles under my feet."

"That's amazing. I'm Julie."

"I'm Ingrid." Her watched beeped. "Time for me to walk now. You go on ahead. Catch some more folks."

It felt good not to be last anymore, I won't lie, but I also didn't feel the need to push. I wanted to finish strong and teach myself to hold back. It only took me 26 marathons to learn. I kept my momentum and my clear head for the remainder of the race. By the end, I could feel my joints ache. Sharp pains shot up my feet all the way to my knees and I wanted to collapse. But the sparkling Colorado River looked so good. I hobbled over to the bank and slowly lowered myself in. David followed behind and sat on a nearby rock.

With my elbows on a rock and the small of my back resting on a rock ledge, I let the calm waters near the shoreline wash over my legs. It was cold, winter cold. I imagined my muscles clenching and relaxing, compressing, letting new blood flow through. My mind went blank. David and I sat quietly for a long time.

"What do you think your time would've been if you hadn't started 15 minutes behind the pack?" He was teasing me, I knew it. I laughed.

"Well, I ran over five hours," I said.

"It doesn't't matter, Julie."

God, he was right. Only one other woman had done 52 in 52. Dana Casanave was her name, and I was following in her footsteps. Time really was irrelevant for this undertaking. No matter if I was last, first, walking, or crawling across the finish. What counted was that I went the distance, crossed the finish line, in a legit 26.2 mile marathon, 52 weeks in a row.

"It doesn't matter," I repeated.

"It doesn't."

But then I thought about my donations page. That did matter.

"David, I don't know how I can get the word out," I said. "I feel like I'm failing."

"No, no," he said. "There is no failing in this. You are doing something incredible and it will all fall into place."

I leaned my head back and closed my eyes. I felt like something had been holding me back. I was waist deep in the freezing Colorado River, and felt a true sense of peace, of calm. Up until this race, I worked to run as fast as I could, to look as good as I could, and to be vocal about my love of running and my cause. But it was a show. Inside, I was still struggling with my father's death and the complex relationship we'd had during my life.

I needed a way to transfer some of that pain, to leave it on the road. I thought that by doing something good for pancreatic cancer awareness and research, I would be able to rest my mind. But maybe it was more personal. I knew I needed to stop worrying about the shallow, trivial things I was so preoccupied with. Who cared if I ran under five hours? Who cared if I wore mascara? My work needed to go beyond all the nonsense. And if I could be myself, stop wearing a mask of pure enthusiasm and glee, I wouldn't be so tired. From now on, I decided, the races and the cause I was racing for were going to be greater than me.

I resolved that day to dedicate all these miles, every race, to people fighting for their lives. The more I cared on an intimate level, the more others would care. The more I recognized them, and the pain their loved ones were going through (pain that I could well relate to), the greater sense of purpose this year of marathoning would have. I was ready to face the next 47 races as an entirely new Julie.

Chapter 12
True to the Cause

A beautiful, spring morning in Santa Monica. I stretched my creaky limbs, pulled myself out of the comforter and got up to look out the window. David had already left for work. On the counter, there was a note. "Have a great day! Love, David." It was a nice way to start a Monday morning and I had a great feeling about the day ahead. I grabbed Jessie, hobbled to Starbucks and ordered a quad-latte. Then I scooped some protein powder I'd brought along, into my cup. This was my drink of choice now.

Work, eat, sleep. Along with those lattes, this was my daily routine. David and I decided that running in between marathons would put undue stress on my body. So instead, I stretched. Recovery was my training, and I was happy for the rest.

208 | Julie Weiss

At the office that day, I greeted my co-workers warmly and with more energy than I had in weeks. I'd started showing off my latest medal to Rod every Monday. I'd have a different race and new bling to show him. He was impressed and became an amazing supporter of my feats. I was so grateful to have his encouragement.

A text from my daughter popped up on my phone.

"Finally, a good Facebook post!" it read.

Ah yes, I recalled. The message I'd posted last night inviting people to share their stories with me. "Ha! Glad you approve!"

I logged into my email. I was stunned. I had more than 500 new messages, and there were more Likes and shares and comments than I'd ever seen before. I was grateful for the attention, but I was even more excited that people wanted to be part of my journey.

Work could wait, I figured. I poured over the testimonials. I felt honored that people were sharing these stories with me.

One email came from a person in Florida who was following a little boy, Denali. He was just 11 years old. The sender included a link to a Facebook page that the boy's mom had set up. The story of his illness started with a stomach ache. His mom, like most parents, thought it was just that—a stomach ache. She told him to sit on the potty for a little bit and see if he felt better.

I remembered saying the same words to my kids when they complained of little cramps. I would tell them that maybe they ate too many cookies.

At the time of the stomach ache, Denali was eight years old. He was sweet, handsome. He loved to play and he loved his siblings. About two weeks after the stomach ache, on the way to school, his older brother tapped his mom on the shoulder. "Mama," he said. "Have you seen Denali's eyes? They're yellow."

I couldn't imagine a small child having to deal with the pain and confusion of this disease. The needles, the poking, the invasive surgeries. The loss of energy and appetite. None of that seemed fair. I couldn't hold him or hug him, but I could run for him. (He would pass away at just 11 years old a month after I dedicated a race to him.) I emailed his mother to let her know—I wanted her to understand that I was another person hoping to make a difference in her son's life. I read the next email.

Kerry's husband Noel was diagnosed April 2011 at 54 years of age with pancreatic cancer. They had booked a family holiday to California, taking the kids to Disney and to renew their wedding vows for their 10th anniversary on a beach in Ventura, CA.

The doctors gave Noel six months to live. Upon the news Noel and Kerry stood outside the hospital just clinging to each other and crying. How could it be? How could she be losing the love of her life? She typed those questions to me, and I understood everything. There wasn't a damn thing either of them or anyone else could do. They decided that renewing their wedding vows was more important than ever. Noel was so sick. Every day he asked how many days until the renewal. August 17th, Noel was released from the hospital 24 hours before they walked down the aisle and pledged their love all over again, till death do us part.

One of Noel's daughters announced she was pregnant. Noel was so thrilled but also so sad he knew he wouldn't be around to see the birth of his first grandchild. Kerry knew Noel didn't have much longer. How do you say goodbye to someone who means everything to you? How can you even think about life without them? She had to tell her children that the angels were coming for daddy, he was tired.

I promised to run for Noel.

Then there was Roberta's note. She lost not only her father to pancreatic cancer, but her uncle and her grandmother as well. Three family members lost to one disease. It was mind-blowing. She worried for her sons and what about her? Her mother was also diagnosed in 2005 and would die in February, 2013.

When Roberta started feeling slightly ill one day, she didn't wait. She went into her doctor and demanded a test be done to determine whether or not pancreatic cancer was brewing inside her. "Like most, I went through a number of tests, most very invasive, before getting diagnosed," Roberta told me.

The doctors told her she was lucky: the tumor was small, it was caught early and if she started treatment immediately, she would have a better chance than most. She started chemotherapy immediately, and also underwent radiation for a short period of time and survived. Because she had lived through the role of survivor and caretaker, Roberta wanted to raise awareness for both. I couldn't believe the strength of this woman. Her mission was to bring hope and joy to anyone affected by the disease. I understood her perspective entirely.

Since he was diagnosed in June 2012, Greg Willard had valiantly fought the disease alongside his wife of 22 years, Laurie, their children Bryce, Shelby, and Weston, as well as many other family members and friends. I had first met Greg at the Pancreatic Cancer Action Network gala in October where he was being honored. It was there that he said to me, "I'll see you at the finish line!" Those words played over in my head as I read his email, thinking of him and his family at their Huntington Beach home; a beautiful picture despite an underlying battle.

Another email: Mitch, a fellow runner, was reaching out to me and thanking me. He, too, had been impacted by this horrible cancer. He wrote, "I am not near 52 marathons in 52 weeks, but I am on my own journey in running, being pushed by thoughts of my dad. Please keep him in mind during one of your strides in the future and please keep up the inspirations you give to everyone." I internally pledged to keep both Mitch and his father in my heart and mind during my next race. We will run together to end this awful disease.

There were too many to read all at once. But I couldn't stop. Christine's mother Carolyn loved Disney World. Carolyn was diagnosed in 2001 at 61 years old. Carolyn loved spending time with her grandchildren, walking the beach, volunteering, traveling, and cooking. She was the best cook. She remembered her mother's incredible lasagna, chocolate chip cookies, and baked stuffed shrimp. Christine wrote and said that the thing she missed most about her mother was that she was such a good listener. Her optimism was unrelenting. She believed she would beat this beast. She knew that time was such a gift; she and Christine appreciated every minute.

I also heard from Kate via Facebook. We share something very personal, very close to our hearts: both of our fathers passed away from pancreatic cancer. She was asking if I could dedicate some of my races to her father, Keith. His birthday had just passed and at the time he would have been 67 years old—still so very young. Kate missed him terribly, a feeling I know well. Although I don't know much about her father, I do know that he was immensely loved by his daughter. And to me, that tells more than enough. I added Kate, Keith and his family to my list. And I kept reading.

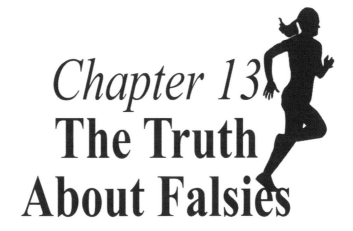

Chapter 13
The Truth
About Falsies

Suddenly, people started to pay attention.

At Grandma's Marathon, number 11, a television news crew surrounded me. The fear I'd once had about speaking in public disappeared when I talked about my mission. I wanted people watching me to feel my positivity and hear the stories of the folks I was now running for. I had my mission story down and could recite my personal narrative in my sleep.

I'm just a mom of two, with a full-time job and on the side, I'm running 52 marathons for pancreatic cancer in honor of my dad and many other good people who have been claimed by this awful disease.

Waiting for my plane on my way back from Minnesota, I made a crucial mistake: I read the comments on a YouTube video about me. An anonymous web troll lambasted me for leaving my two kids at home while I ran. "But that's not the case," I said aloud to my phone. "My kids are older. They have lives of their own." My son was 24, my daughter 19—and in Europe, studying abroad!

"Julie, what's wrong?" David had seen me scowling. I showed him the post. "Well tell that woman the truth! You lock your kids in cages down the basement while you're away."

I groaned. David laughed at his own joke.

By this point, he was filming everything, with the idea of creating a mini-series about my "52 For You" effort (the name we had started giving to my marathon quest, since the outpouring of personal stories). The narrator wasn't David. Instead, he introduced a new character to the story. A purple stuffed animal, a felt, amorphous blob with googly eyeballs who recapped every painstaking detail. We called him Thing.

To make the stuffed thing come to life, David used a cracking, high-pitched voice. "Hey there race fans," he would say behind the camera. Sometimes the creature would speak from our apartment, using my race medals as a back drop. The camera would focus in on his lifeless, unmoving body.

David thought it was so bad it was good. I thought it was just plain bad. It continued, race after race and in our home. I tried to tune him out, and the noise of the rest of the world, because Kona was next. Kona, the place I felt most like myself. I would carry my new momentum all the way to Hawaii and then be renewed, again, by the air and ocean. Hopefully, I wouldn't have to carry an amorphous purple blob with me.

In Kona, it was quiet. News crews did not greet us at the airport and reporters weren't texting me nonstop. After a few races that demanded a lot from my budding public persona, I was glad to have a rest.

But Thing continued to pester me.

"David there is too much Thing," I told him in private. "The race director from the Kona Marathon wanted some video and all we have is this stupid purple thing, everywhere! Get rid of it."

"I think it's funny," he said. And, to be fair, it was kind of funny. But it's not the type of thing you can give to race or media outlets.

"David, you are a very creative man, a funny guy," I said. "But this is not *Sesame Street*."

I think that's the last we heard of Thing. RIP.

I was happy on my quest and felt a sense of peace in this beautiful place. I was already on the 12th marathon, and nothing could stop me now. At the start, it was dark. We took off to the sound of a horn, blown by a man in traditional Hawaiian garb. On the course, I mentally called out to my dad. Hawaii was where I initiated the changes in my life that had led me back here. I wanted to share that memory with him. As usual, we hustled through the airport. David trailed just behind me rattling off a checklist.

"You have the foam roller in your carry-on?"

"Yup."

"You have an empty water bottle?"

"Yup."

"You drank your whole protein smoothie?"

"I did."

At airport security, I needed to be patted down. I'd decided at that time to stop getting myself radiated by the x-ray machines, and just have someone check me over instead. I'd grown used to the inconveniences of air travel. I stepped to the side and waited for the female TSA agent. She looked me up and down. I was wearing my purple tank top and compression tights—this look had become my uniform.

She patted me down, the backs of her hand gently sliding

up and down my sides. Then, she leaned in uncomfortably close. "You know, you got a bulge," she said. She pointed at my breast.

"Wait, what?"

"It's probably nothing, but I wanted to let you know."

"They're fake, maybe that's what you're feeling?"

"Maybe, but that left one is a heck of a lot bigger than the right. You don't have anything in there, right?"

"Nope."

She looked me up and down. I raised my eyebrows and gave her my most innocent, "no I'm not smuggling drugs in my boobs" face.

"Okay you're good. Maybe get that checked out."

"Thanks," I said.

I appreciated the TSA agent's concern, but I didn't have time to go to doctors. I figured as long as I felt okay, I would be okay. That night in the shower, I did my own check. The agent was right, my left breast was much bigger than my right. Now, most women have size variances, but this was not right. It was hardened, like a rock under my skin. And the sides poked out.

Still, I had a race to run. But during Leadville, my chest hurt. Not my heart or my lungs, but my boob. My breast. I started paying attention to it—was it a different size? Was it really shaped like that? Had it always looked like that? Something was wrong. I promised I would get it checked out, I just wasn't sure when.

Besides the boob thing, I felt pretty good that race. You run up the side of a mountain, well past 11,000 feet at mile nine—and then there's 2,000 more feet of incline. David met me around mile 10, and I tapped the brakes, coming to a halt. "We can walk," I said. "God help me."

He didn't really ask many questions, just meandered along the mountainside. "I was tired at mile one," I said. "And my iPod is out of juice. It's done."

I'd loaded my trusty iPod with a bunch of different music. Anything from Rage Against the Machine to Mary Poppins. I used music for any race that allowed headphones. But now, it was dead. I tried my best, telling David and the spectators around me that I didn't need music, I would just sing my way to the finish. But the few notes of "Over the Rainbow" that I could manage left me gasping for air. We were indeed way up high.

David pointed ahead and asked if I could see the tallest mountain in the Mosquito Range. That was the next stop. I nodded. I knew. Dammit, I was tired.

I walked a little. Actually, I walked a lot. I ran my first 30-minute mile of my life and had no shame about it. Climbing that ascent, getting up to 13.1K feet above sea level killed my legs, but doing it, conquering it, and running back down was unlike any marathon accomplishment I've ever had. David was there at the foot of the switchbacks, camera in hand.

"I'm still smiling," I said. "And now I'm gonna get going, because we have a plane to catch."

Number 14, on July 4, was the Foot Traffic Flat Marathon in Oregon followed four days later by the Missoula Marathon.

Another week, another race. My chest still didn't feel quite right, but I wasn't about to let it slow me down. I figured when I got back from the Light at the End of the Tunnel, a hidden gem of a marathon in Seattle that starts with a two-mile tunnel and ends with amazing finish line food, I'd see a doctor. I was pretty sure I knew what it was—one of my implants was out of place. Maybe it was a result of all the running. I didn't tell anyone but David about my discomfort. I didn't want my new social followers to know, or to think I was complaining. Most of them had someone they loved in tremendous pain. Mine—something likely caused by a cosmetic surgery—seemed trite by comparison. So, onward I went, wearing extra-support sports bras and hoping like hell no one could see my lopsided chest.

We went off to Seattle. The race was supposed to be fast. It literally goes through a mountain, in a pitch-black tunnel that lasts for 2.4 miles. I was spooked, for sure. At the start line, every runner had a headlamp on and joked about ghosts lurking in the corners, or murderers just waiting for us in the dark.

David was back in action with his camera. He started the race with me, trying to get way ahead so he could film me coming from the darkness. He pulled ahead, and I followed the light. About 50 yards in, you can't see anything around you but other headlamps bobbing up and down. But you can almost make out a small speck of light leading you to the other side. It should've been a symbol of hope, maybe a metaphor for the remaining races, but instead it was just immediate relief: I needed to get to that light fast. My breathing was ragged, my body felt unfamiliar in the dark. I was afraid I would trip someone, or someone might trip me. But the bodies around me continued straight ahead, each one of us following the other light, making our way carefully to the other side.

It was easy at first. The flat course with a slow, generous decline gave confidence. After some treacherous races with mountains and heat, The Tunnel was a well-deserved break. I found my stride and my regular pace and felt good, for a while.

David caught me coming out of the tunnel and said he knew

222 | Julie Weiss

how to meet me at other places. He was going to go backwards through the tunnel, once all the runners were through and I would see him soon, he said. Of course, he was still recording. What I didn't know, and what I wouldn't know until the end of the race, is that David took off into the tunnel and ran about a half a mile by himself. Then, with two miles still to go, his head lamp—the one I gave to him when I made it through—ran out of battery power. Alone, in a suffocating darkness, he waded through the pitch black. It was musty inside and each footstep echoed. Any other noise – drops of water, strange and undetectable booms—made him jump. "Creepy," he would say later. But at the time, he couldn't describe the panic he felt. He just kept running, determined to meet me at the spot he had planned.

And when he made it, and I made it to him, I just waved him off.

"How's it going?" He asked.

"It's fine." I didn't want to stop and chat. I wanted to run. I didn't ask how he was or look to see that his hands were shaking holding the camera. I just ran by, shrugging him off. I didn't understand why I was taking my frustrations out on David. Not only did it hurt David, but it hurt me too.

It was my mom, who never understood why I got the implants in the first place, who convinced me to see a doctor. I explained that I just didn't feel good about my chest after having Samantha. Two babies can really deflate things, if you know what I mean. I thought that maybe because she was a modern dancer, she didn't understand the allure of breasts. But to me, to be a true California girl, boobs helped. Or at least it seemed that way in my twenties.

But now, they were backfiring.

The MRI confirmed that my right breast implant ruptured.

"How?" I asked the doctor. The bulge was pressing against the thin hospital gown I wore on the table. I hugged my arms over my chest.

"Well, it could've been the running and extra stress on your body, or it could've been a recent mammogram."

"Well, is it serious?"

"Your breast formed a capsular contraction to keep the silicon away from your body—which is what the body should do. But that's why your breast has gotten bigger and hardened."

If this had happened to anyone else, it would've been simple: get them out and replace them or leave it and recover from the surgery. I tried to explain this to the doctor.

"Julie, they need to come out," he said. "We need to clean

up the silicon that leaked."

"Can it wait? Maybe until next year?"

"No."

"How long is the recovery?"

"Three weeks."

"And that's without getting them replaced?"

"Right."

"Can it wait two weeks?"

He sighed. We put an appointment on the calendar, so I could get through marathons 17 and 18.

Driving to work after the San Francisco Marathon (#18), with my legs aching and cramping, I thought back to my training schedule before the 52. I used to run to work. Six miles to the gym near my office where I would shower, change and enter the workplace bright and shiny and ready to tackle the day. Today, I was battling traffic, rushing to make it in on time. I'd overslept, missed an interview with a reporter, which I rescheduled for later in the day. That meant skipping lunch and finding a quiet place to talk to the journalist while I crammed a protein bar in my face. Plus, the bulge in my breast would not be ignored for much longer.

Worse than any pain, my mind couldn't wrap itself around losing the implants. It may sound strange to men or to women who have never had them, but they had become a part of who I was. Would I still feel sexy without them? Would I look good in clothes? I planned on buying all new tops and new bras. But even worse than what it would do to my self-image, was my mission: I would have to spend three weeks not running; three weeks of missing races. I'd planned ahead, though, and gave myself a little cushion. I had the Tahoe Triple on my list, which meant I'd need to run three marathons in three days. I would make up the distance, but man, I dreaded that weekend.

I dreaded this weekend, too. We flew to Las Vegas, Nevada on Friday for The Extraterrestrial Full Moon Midnight Marathon. The course was miles outside the city, in an isolated part of the desert. It started at midnight and ran around the infamous Area 51, a supposed holding place for aliens captured by the government.

I'd chosen this race, not just because it worked for my schedule. The very idea of holding a race in this strange, spooky location made it a singular experience. I was ready for something different. This could be fun—although that probably wouldn't be a word to describe what living with me was like.

By this point, I felt myself slowly turning into someone I did not recognize. I was cranky all the time, preoccupied by my physical pain, and anxious at the start of every week. A high would come immediately after a marathon, but by the next morning, I would dive headfirst into a scary low—knowing I would have to do it all over again the following week. This process that had me dancing and singing in the kitchen at the very idea of it, was now a great struggle. I never thought of how much grit I would need to do it all. I found inspiration from those I was running for and felt silly complaining about a busted implant and sore quads compared to those battling pancreatic cancer, but it was hard, and my energy and hormones were in the toilet.

I was strong, with thick muscles and sturdy bones. I never thought my breasts would be what held me back. Then again, perhaps an exploding implant was really a blessing in disguise. I just had to make it down the Extraterrestrial Highway and then I'd get a brief respite.

Race organizers arranged for eight busses to transport the runners from Las Vegas to the course. We loaded the bus in our glowing gear and head lamps and traveled out of the city, leaving the bright lights behind us. It's amazing how dark it is as soon as you leave Las Vegas. The city is like a vast beam of light, with miles of blackness around it. I didn't like running in the dark.

"Ugh,' I said, looking out at the blackness that had swallowed up our bus.

David, sitting next to me, said nothing. He took my hand and squeezed. He knew that this would be a challenge for me.

Running in the dark is unsettling. I don't even like running in the rain. At home in sunny Santa Monica, on the seldom occasion when fog rolls in, I'll sulk until it burns off. But here, in the dead of night, I knew there was no chance of sun for hours. I would have to rely on the moon.

"It'll be brighter in a few hours," David said.

"Sure," I said. "It'll go from pitch black to really black."

The moon did illuminate the inky sky, but there was not much to see. As we started, headlamps bounced off scraggly Joshua trees. Their twisted branches made eerie shadows along the side of the road. What happened at Area 51 is still unknown. While I don't believe in aliens running around the Nevada desert, the highly classified property is spooky to say the least. What went on beyond the "No Trespassing" signs? As the miles rolled along, I fell into a dream state, like sleep-running. The air was crisp and dry, and it felt like it was getting colder—a shiver ran up my spine. Stopping to walk here was out of the question—I might be abducted by aliens! I plodded along, allowing my eyes to close for moments at a time.

I was alone. There was no one around me to keep me

228 | Julie Weiss

awake, or talk to, or even follow. I wondered if I was the only living thing around for miles. My eyelids fluttered open, then closed, then open again. A thin shadow—an outline of a body was lumbering down the road.

It moved clumsily but quickly, hunched slightly at the shoulders with a dragging gait. Was there actually an alien on the course? Or more likely, some idiot dressed as an alien? It looked like it could be human. My pace slowed.

The dark figure continued to approach.

It had a flashlight and was shining it in my direction. I closed my eyes, ready to surge ahead. Outrunning it was my only choice. Hopefully aliens couldn't run faster than nine-minute miles.

"Julie?"

It was David.

"Oh," I gasped, my heart filling with relief. "David. Oh my God."

"Not an alien," he laughed.

I took his neck in my hands and pulled him close and kissed him. I had never been so grateful for him, so happy to see him.

"How far did you run to get out here?" I asked.

"Just eight miles or so from the finish."

"Thank you."

"C'mon, I'll run with you for a bit."

We took off. I still felt like I could fall asleep on my feet, but I felt safe. David ran along next to me in silence. The sun started to rise. In the distance, I could see its orange face coming over the mountains. The sky lit up in blues and yellows. By 6:00 a.m., I was less than two miles from the finish. David had run ahead, getting ready for me to cross the line and preparing my warm clothes. It would've been my father's 77th birthday. I thought maybe he was lighting up the sky for me, helping me through the darkness once again.

"That was awful," I said at the finish. A man next to me smiled. Unbeknownst to me, he was the race director. Don't get me wrong, it was great marathon, I just don't do well without any sleep. I left the full moon marathon with a full heart though. I had a new appreciation for David and I felt extremely grateful he was there for me. He's always there for me.

But with the E.T. Marathon out of the way, I had another challenge. The boob surgery. More than fearing the surgery itself, I was scared I wouldn't be able to get back on track. And I had other worries too.

Traveling back from Las Vegas, I wrote a blog that no one ever saw.

7/28- About to get exploded boobs out.

Sitting here on the plane, trying to smile knowing I am having my breasts taken out in just over a week, it's really hard.

I want to be the positive person that I am and focus on all the good, because there really is a lot but it's so hard. Everything is bothering me right now.

For someone who has as always held up a certain image: blonde hair, boobs. I know I care too much about how I look. It's all ego. There is so much more. What a crazy experience this is. I am so sad, so devasted I cry every night.

I hate having this toxic stuff inside of me. Get it out!

I wanted to post this, to ask for support from my friends and followers, but I couldn't. I kept reminding myself that this journey was about more than me.

After the surgery, I was sore. I didn't think it was going to be so bad, but now I was looking down at my scarred skin. It hurt like hell. Drains and stitches and raw, pink skin erupted out of my chest. I was disfigured and horrified.

Yes, I cared about appearance too much. Why couldn't I shake the insecurity that I'd carried with me all my life? No matter how much makeup I used, what clothes I bought, I wasn't satisfied. My eyelashes were never long and beautiful enough (so I got fake ones), my hair wasn't thick enough (so I blew it out), and I rarely felt sexy (probably because of the criticism I felt as a child).

Of course, earlier in my life, I used the attention of men to boost myself up. If they looked at me with desire, then I must have the charms they want. But until my breasts literally exploded, I never questioned why I felt the way I did about my looks.

Sitting on my couch, Jessie by my side, the pump draining infected looking fluids from my chest, I wondered why I would go to such great lengths to make myself feel whole. And what would happen now, with a lopsided chest that couldn't be remedied for months.

I couldn't help but remember my father's old insults. Mostly, he'd complain about my weight. He was a critical man who valued beauty. His wife, my mother, was slender—a totally different body type from me. I was tall, like him, and built with curves—hips and breasts—even before augmentation. I wanted to cancel that voice in my head. That voice, which I call Negative Nelly, parrots some of the worst things my father ever said. *You are ugly*, she would say. *There are so many people prettier and faster than you. You are old, you'll never amount to anything.* What a bitch

Nelly is. I assured myself that my father didn't mean what he said, and that he couldn't have known the damage it caused to my self-esteem. I felt guilty, with a healthy dose of self-loathing, for being shallow enough to think of my looks, when I was supposed to be raising money for people battling a lethal form of cancer.

David assured me that he loved my body, no matter what. But when he came in to hug me, my first instinct was to yell, "don't touch me." I felt damaged. He tried to help, and I wanted to let him nurse me back to health, but I couldn't let him near my scars at first.

A week after the surgery, the meds wore off and so did some of the sadness. I could walk around with ease and no pain. And something changed: I felt like a badass. I'd made it through a horrendous surgery, I'd run with exploding implants, and I'd completed 19 marathons in 19 weeks. In two weeks, I would be back on the marathon course.

I started experimenting with the false boobs the plastic surgeon gave to me. They were little silicon inserts, like external implants, that looked like chicken cutlets. I decided, to feel more confident, I would wear them for news interviews and appearances.

"David," I said while walking around with them in our apartment, "you're on boob check."

I wanted him to alert me if one of the "cutlets" were sticking out of my bra. We laughed together. It felt like the first time we'd laughed since Kona.

"Julie, you look great," he said. He also reminded me that losing 10 pounds of fat would help me run a minute faster. "I don't think those were quite 10 pounds, but I bet you anything you'll shave some seconds off your time."

I laughed. "Thanks, David. Maybe now I'll PR."

We both breathed a sigh of relief. David wasn't thrilled with his new boob inspector job, but he would do it. We wondered if we needed a special sign if one of the falsies was flying around, and we settled on a subtle point to the chest area.

Given my new breast stress, a few times I found myself throwing my new foam boobs at David. To which, he would throw them back at me. We were having boob fights. I thanked him for being so helpful through the process.

"I feel kind of awesome," I said. That week of pain and guilt and shame let me process something that always deeply troubled me. I looked in the mirror in the bathroom and took the little inserts out. I stared at my chest. It looked deflated, but kind of beautiful. I was proud of myself for getting the surgery, for picking myself up after feeling so down, and for continuing on. "You are strong," I said to myself. "You are powerful."

Kauai—another one of my all-time favorite races—was the next on the list. With my new chicken cutlets and confidence, I was ready for my comeback. Still, I touched my chest the whole way, making sure nothing was falling out. I kept catching strangers' eyes and wondering if they were staring at my boobs. Or maybe they knew that I'd just had my implants taken out.

C'mon Hawaii, heal me.

I needed the land to renew me again. But instead of the beaches answering my wishes, I reminded myself that I had the power. And I did. Once 20 was done, I started thinking about 21. Mahalo Kauai.

Chapter 14
The Marathon That Almost Never Was

A loud and low flyover by two V-22 Ospreys.

A rousing speech with lots of inspiring, martial talk about being "mission ready" and "assaulting the District," punctuated by thousands of full-throated "Ooh-rahs."

And for good measure, a blast from a howitzer.

Yes, just as they are second to none in recruiting slogans, dress uniforms and mystique-building—not to mention combat— the United States Marines Corps sure knows how to kick off a marathon. Like the other 25,000 runners in the field of the 2012

Marine Corps Marathon, I was totally excited by the time the Ospreys—part jet, part helicopter—roared overhead, followed shortly by the deep thud of the cannon that echoed across the field near
the Pentagon and signaled the start of the race, the fifth largest
marathon in the U.S.

And yet, there was something even more powerful and
more ominous than all that Marine energy and firepower hanging
over this event: A massive hurricane that was barreling up the East
Coast at the very moment we were set to run through Washington,
D.C. It was expected to make landfall the following night, somewhere in New Jersey.

The storm already had a name—one that would become infamous throughout the East Coast before long: Superstorm Sandy.

As a lifelong Cali girl, I know bizarre weather. Mudslides,
fires and earthquakes periodically punctuate our picture-perfect
days. But what do I know from hurricanes? As it turned out, I
would become all too familiar with this one. While nothing compared to the devastation wrought by this storm across the Eastern
Seaboard, Sandy would become another enormous obstacle in my
52-marathon quest leading David and I on a cross-country travel
odyssey that may have been as draining as any of the actual marathons I ran.

Of course, I didn't realize this at the start of Marine Corps. I was too busy being distracted by all these sharp-looking Marines at the water stops, crisply administering our fluid replenishment needs. I was also taking in the awe-inspiring scenery of our nation's capital—my first visit there—and the warm camaraderie of my fellow competitors. The Marine Corps Marathon is called "The People's Marathon" for a reason. There's no prize money here; no Olympians or professional racers. Although the vast majority of the runners are neither present or retired service men or women, the winners are often fast young runners from the military (ours or others—a lot of other nations send their competitive service teams).

Fast, I was not. I was nursing a knee injury that morning. All right, "injury" might be too strong a word. "Off-ness" might a better term. My right leg just didn't feel like it was firing at 100 percent. It was one of the nagging, garden variety overuse ailments I would battle for a good chunk of the 52 marathon/52week challenge. But because I didn't feel like I was running smoothly, I ended up walking much of the first half. Then at around 10 and a half miles into the race—along the Hains Point peninsula that juts into the Potomac—we entered what organizers call "The Blue Mile."

Here, for an entire mile, the road is lined with photos of

U.S. servicemen and women killed in combat since 2001. The photos, framed in deep blue like the field of the American flag, are posted along the road every few feet. It's one shining young face after another; one more father, son, mother or daughter, who never returned, and like many of the other participants in the marathon, I was in tears halfway through.

But the Blue Mile had another, unexpected effect on me. It made me think that whatever discomfort or pain I was feeling in this—an undertaking of my own choosing—and whatever sacrifices I was making to pursue this quixotic dream of mine, it paled compared to the ultimate sacrifice made by these heroes, and the loss and suffering their families endured.

I suppose at that moment also, some inner Marine Corps drill instructor in me—and believe me, I didn't know until that point that I even had one—thrust his rock-jawed visage into my brain and basically said. "Weiss! Stop screwing around and get your ass in gear! This is a race, not a walk in the park. You got a boo-boo? Suck it up and start running."

Which is exactly what I did. I picked up the pace, and the discomfort in my knee vanished, as if it was responding to an order. It's interesting how every once in a while, the cure for a running ailment is more running, and this thought, plus my first glimpses of the Washington Monument, the Capitol Building, and the Pentagon, kept my attention.

Oh, and I can't forget the Magic Marine Beans. At mile 19, the Marines were handing out energy beans: Similar to the shots, blocks and chews that are commonly used by distance runners, these beans had some electrolytes, carbs, and apparently, a heavy dose of caffeine. I picked up my pace some more, forgot about my knee, and was all fired up. I kept yelling "We got this!" which was becoming my motto. I hooted and hollered even more than normal, and when my iPod ran out of power, I started singing out loud.

Yes, I know this sounds sacrilegious to serious runners—but the truth is, I wasn't running hard. I was running long. Week after week. It was as much a mental challenge as it was physiological. And so, if I decide to start singing, sing out loud *Europe's* "The Final Countdown," who cares?

As much as my nonstop talking could annoy some runners, these kinds of good-natured histrionics, I've learned, can be contagious: I think I even heard a couple of the runners near me start humming along to the song.

On the flip side, sometimes the spectators made me laugh. I recall chuckling at one sign I saw later in the race, "Run Faster, Hurricane Sandy is Right Behind You."

Ha-ha, I thought. That's funny.

The marathon finishes by the U.S. Marine Corps War Memorial—a/k/a the Iwo Jima Memorial. Seeing the iconic image of the Marines raising the flag was as uplifting and moving as the Blue Mile. I got my finish line photo taken—with the memorial behind me—and headed back to our hotel. I called David, who had not accompanied me on this race, and although even-keeled as always, I could tell that he felt a sense of urgency as I navigated the crowded post-race streets of Arlington.

"Julie, I wouldn't dawdle at the hotel," he said. "You can't miss this flight. I'm even thinking maybe you should try and re-book an earlier one."

"Why?" I said. Over the previous six months, I'd become quite the blasé traveler, in some ways. I figured there was always another flight to Los Angeles. Maybe not this time, though.

"They may start cancelling flights because of that storm. They're saying this is going to be bad."

Oh yeah, that storm. I thought of the sign held by the spectator, and now it didn't seem quite as amusing.

I looked overhead. Ominous dark clouds were beginning to form.

"Got it," I said, still buzzed by post-marathon endorphins.

"I'll resist the temptation to order champagne from room service and take a long, hot bath."

David didn't miss a beat. "Take a shower instead, and have a drink on the plane."

I hustled back to the hotel, showered, packed quickly and got over to the airport as soon as I could. Reagan National was packed with nervous flyers, many of them of them finishers like me, wearing their official Marine Corps Marathon jackets and hats, while casting nervous glances at the schedule boards, expecting to see the words "Delayed" or, worse, "See Agent."

Fortunately, I boarded without a problem, and flew home without incident. But I did hear later that David's concerns were well founded: Apparently, they started cancelling flights soon after we'd departed.

As I was jetting across the country, the New York Times of Monday, October 29 was hitting streets and screens with this alarming headline: "NORTHEAST BRACES FOR DEADLY SURGE AND LASHING WIND."

At 7:30 p.m. that night, I was shaking off some jet lag back at work in Los Angeles—the storm slammed into Atlantic City, New Jersey, with winds up to 80 miles per hour.

New York City was right in its cross hairs: As an official

report on the storm's impact later explained, the angle of approach put the five boroughs in the worst possible position. The winds that had been blowing south—essentially towards the storm—had shifted northwest as the storm made landfall. This helped give Sandy a push; and propelled the storm's enormous surge, and its punishing waves, directly towards the city.

The result? The report, published later by the city, ticked off the staggering statistics in the five boroughs alone:

* *43 deaths, 6,500 patients evacuated from hospitals and nursing homes...*

* *Nearly 90,000 buildings in the inundation zone... 1.1 million New York City children unable to attend school for a week...*

* *Close to 2 million people without power...*

* *11 million travelers affected daily...*

* *$19 billion in damage...*

The spectacular damage stirred up by the storm included a record, 32-foot wave that struck the tip of Manhattan, flooding power-stations and subway tunnels. Entire neighborhoods were severely damaged, and in one apocalyptic scene, 110 houses in the seaside Queens community of Breezy Point were consumed in an out-of-control fire.

Like many across the rest of the United States, we watched

much of this unfold on TV. While my first reaction was concern and sympathy for the people living in New York, I must admit that my second reaction was a bit more selfish.

"Holy shit," I thought. "I'm supposed to be running a marathon there on Sunday!"

The New York City Marathon, scheduled for that Sunday, Nov. 1, quickly became an unwelcome part of the Sandy story.

A front-page story in the tabloid New York Post showed a photo of three generators in Central Park. "As hundreds of thousands of Big Apple residents suffer in homes left without power by Hurricane Sandy," the story blared, "two massive generators are being run 24/7 in Central Park — to juice a media tent for Sunday's New York City Marathon."

An accompanying editorial boasted the headline, "Marathon is Power Mad."

Hundreds of thousands of New Yorkers huddle in the dark each night after the most devastating storm in city history — while two massive generators chug away in Central Park and a third sits idle waiting to power a media center during Sunday's NYC Marathon.

Like hell.

Those generators could power 400 homes on Staten Island

or the Rockaways or any storm-wracked neighborhood in the city certain to be suffering the after-effects of Hurricane Sandy on Sunday morning.

Shouldn't they come first? Shouldn't the race just be canceled?

Damned straight.

While the pugnacious editorial was really an attack on the Post's favorite target of the time—Mayor Michael Bloomberg—the story quickly spread and spurred outrage, not only in New York, but even out here in Los Angeles where I soon found myself debating my participation with colleagues at work, as well as on social media. Should the marathon be held or not? To be fair, if I was without power on Staten Island or the Rockaways that week, and I saw those massive generators being earmarked for the media covering a foot race, I'd be ticked off too. That said, the sentiment was far from unanimous. Many people in New York besides Mayor Bloomberg, wanted to see it held, arguing that it would be a symbol of resilience and toughness in a city that had bounced back from the 9-11 terrorist attacks and could damn well rise up from the blow dealt by this storm, too.

I found myself tap-tapping away on my phone or laptop, defending the mayor and the New York Road Runners and those, like me, who wanted to run that Sunday. But I was conflicted. I even discussed it with my therapist. "Am I doing the right thing?"

Her response helped me formulate a fist-pounding, flag-waving blog post:

"I'm going to New York to show the American people that we're strong even in the face of chaos," I wrote. "Let's show them that nothing is going to stop us. We are determined to do this as part of the fight against pancreatic cancer."

In response, I got a lot of "you go, girl" and "Julie for President" comments. But others felt differently. "There's plenty of other places where you can be running and raising money this weekend," someone wrote. "Right now, the people in New York have bigger fish to fry."

Again, I felt conflicted. But I still had to prepare. My weeks during the marathon streak had followed a somewhat predictable and structured fashion—or as predictable and structured as I can get.

To this day, people continue to tell me how amazing I was to be able to run a marathon once a week for a year. That's exactly the word I'd use, too. It was truly amazing that I actually got my act together to do it. To me, the marathons were the simplest part of the process. Not "easy"—a marathon always takes effort and determination, even if you're having fun running it. But in terms of complications, crossing the finish line was usually not the issue. Getting to the start line? Another story. I'm not the most organized person in the world. As I look back on those weeks in 2012-13—the weeks punctuated by weekend marathons—it's a blur of Starbucks visits (the baristas at my local, on Main Street in Santa Monica started making the quad latte the minute I walked in); social media (I worked it, posting constantly, thanking donors, writing my blogs, and watching my followers grow from zero to 7,000 at that point); trying to stay focused on my job. Rod was so forgiving, but it was understandable that his patience was running short. Any more missed days, the fear of being fired loomed.

Oh, and packing. Or unpacking, depending on how you look at it. Organized chaos is a polite description of my apartment at that point. It was basically a mountain of clothes in a corner, foam boobs everywhere, laundry waiting to be washed, or repacked into my purple Marathon Goddess travel bag. This was a gift for me from a woman whose husband had died of pancreatic cancer. As a way to support my efforts, she made me this beautiful carry-on bag. It had an over-the-shoulder strap and the words Marathon Goddess stitched on the side.

I also had a matching purple, roll-on suitcase; one of those four-wheel jobs that allow you to just glide through airport terminals. That was a gift too—my neighbors had seen me one morning, frantically trying to catch a plane while schlepping my old suitcase through the parking lot to my car. They were like, "Oh my God, Julie, stop it. You're going to be traveling every week? You need a serious suitcase."

Besides helping me travel in comfort and style, the support from good folks like this kept me thinking that what I was doing was worthwhile. People were connecting to it; people were behind it.

Well, maybe not everybody.

There were some haters out there—runners, even, who hated the idea that the marathon would be held while so many people were in dire straits. "They need to take care of the city!" was one comment I got.

As a people pleaser, I liked to think that everyone is with me, everyone is behind me—especially in this crazy marathon adventure of mine. Hey, who doesn't want to support the fight against cancer? But now I felt like I was in the hot seat. Because I had written on my blog about my commitment to running New York, a few L.A. reporters called me. They asked me if I had mixed feelings. I did. But I was still going. I could only hope it was the right

248 | Julie Weiss

decision.

I fretted for the entirety of the flight. When we arrived, David grabbed us a cab. On our way to our hotel, in midtown Manhattan, the driver was telling us how bad things were. And I'm in the back seat, thinking "I'm a terrible person!"

It got worse as we drove into the city. I saw lines for gas that seemed miles long. I saw the crane dangling from a tower under construction on 57th Street, seemingly hanging by a thread 1,000 feet high. The crane, which had snapped during the storm, had become an instant tourist attraction (although one best observed from a distance, as the police had the streets directly under the building cordoned off). Elsewhere, people were on the streets, restaurants and bars filled, and the city still pulsed with energy. While there were no signs of panic or despair in the faces I saw—hey it was New York, after all—you knew that this wasn't business as usual in the Big Apple. I really began to second guess my decision to run.

"Are you sure this is the right thing to do?" I asked David. "What if we get rocks thrown at us on the course?"

We arrived at our hotel and got on line to check in. The registration desk was adjacent to the bar. While we didn't notice it at first, the TVs mounted over the bar had just broken into regular programming with a special announcement. The Mayor had issued a statement about Sunday's marathon and a live press briefing was about to take place.

"While holding the race would not require diverting resources from the recovery effort, it is clear that it has become the source of controversy and division," Michael Bloomberg said in the statement, released jointly with Mary Wittenberg, then president of the New York Road Runners. "The marathon has always brought our city together and inspired us with stories of courage and determination. We would not want a cloud to hang over the race or its participants, and so we have decided to cancel it. We cannot allow a controversy over an athletic event – even one as meaningful as this – to distract attention away from all the critically important work that is being done to recover from the storm and get our city back on track."

At the briefing, an ashen-faced Wittenberg was joined by deputy mayor Howard Wolfson, who acknowledged that the race had become "divisive and controversial" and "a distraction" to storm-relief efforts.

We heard a commotion in the bar area, as people reacted to the news. I looked at David, and he looked at me. "Oh, shit..." I thought. What had transpired now? The crane fell? A fire? More blackouts?

We went over to the bar. "What happened?" David asked.

"They cancelled the marathon," someone responded.

David knew just what I needed at that moment.

"One Bacardi with Coke, please," he told the bartender. David saw the shocked, disoriented expression on my face and quickly amended his order. "Better make it a double," he said. "And I'll have an iced tea."

Dazed, discouraged and jet-lagged, I sipped my drink. By the time the glass was half empty it was clear what I needed to do. "I've just got to find another marathon, David," I said. "There's got to be one somewhere this Sunday that we can reach by plane tomorrow."

There was—and it turned out to be a heckuva lot closer to home than I realized. I texted a buddy of mine at the L.A. Road Runners, who had been helping me with the registration process of the 52 and doing some hand holding. "There's one in Santa Clarita," he responded. "Practically a hometown race!"

Santa Clarita, a bucolic pocket of northern Los Angeles County: I vaguely knew there was a marathon there, but I hadn't realized it was the same day as New York.

I immediately went on the website and called the number

listed, which was the office of the special events department of the City of Santa Clarita. After I was transferred a couple times, the marathon race director, Patrick Downing, got on the phone.

"Pat here, can I help you?"

He probably didn't know what hit him.

"Hi-this-is-Julie-Weiss-I'm-from-Santa-Monica-and-I'm-in-New-York-and-the-marathon-is-cancelled-and-I-have-this-streak-going-and-I'm-going-to-lose-it-and-all-the-cancer-patients-will-be-disappointed-if-I-can't-do-another-marathon-this-weekend-and-I-know-it's-last-minute-but-is-there-any-chance-you-can-please-please-please-let-me-in-your-race?"

That's really how it sounded. I don't think I even took a breath.

"Don't worry, Julie," Pat said. "You're more than welcome to run with us. When do you think you'll get home?"

I told him that we would be catching a morning flight from JFK, and we would drive right up to Santa Clarita from LAX.

"Great, we'll see you at the number pick up tomorrow," he said. "Just ask for me, when you get here. Travel safe, and again, don't worry. We've got you covered."

I wanted to hug him. What a relief!

On a Saturday, it would take us a little over a half hour on the 405 from LAX to Santa Clarita. Now, all I had to do was fly three thousand miles.

David booked a flight home from JFK for the next morning, at 7 a.m. I still couldn't believe I was making plans to leave New York almost as soon as I'd arrived. "David," I said. "Can we go see the finish line?"

We walked up to the park from our hotel, past barricades and signs set up for the marathon that had yet to be taken down. We saw the infamous generators. We saw the grandstands that, on a better day, would have been filled with cheering spectators. We saw the finish line. I insisted on jogging across it, in my street clothes. I had to squeeze through some fencing to get to it. What were they going to do, at this point, I figured? Arrest me?

"Okay," I said. "Let the record show I did cross the finish line of the New York City Marathon."

That night, a cousin of David's who lived in New York visited us. He had something to show me: A copy of the New York Road Runners magazine—the annual Marathon edition—with a story about me.

"A collector's item," David said, dryly.

I could only shake my head.

I also left behind thousands of other out-of-town runners

in a similar predicament. Because none of them were trying to keep a crazy every-weekend marathon streak alive, they looked at other options. It was later reported that many of my fellow visiting marathoners got involved in post-Sandy volunteer efforts around the city that weekend and on Non-Marathon Sunday, an estimated 2,000 runners would run loops of Central Park in an unofficial alternate to the cancelled race. It was planned quickly on Friday and Saturday, on social media. On the sunny, cold morning of No-vember 4, some of them actually did run the marathon distance, 26.2—four loops of Central Park (the original course of the NYC Marathon from 1970-75.)

Later, I wondered if I should have done that, too. But ob-sessiveness and stubbornness are part of a marathoner's make up. I had a cause, I had people who were cheering me on and support-ing me with donations, and I just couldn't allow myself to stop the streak now.

I mulled all this, as I sat sullenly on the flight back to Los Angeles. I was exhausted; my internal clock was completely screwed up. Was I on Eastern Time, Pacific Time, Hurricane Sandy Time? I had no idea. My right knee, the same one that had bothered me during Marine Corps the previous Sunday, picked that time to start throbbing again. Great, I thought. Now I won't be able to even run this 5,000-person Santa Clarita race.

At that point, I remembered one of my many new Facebook friends, Ashley Anderson. She was 26 at the time and had been diagnosed with Stage 4 pancreatic cancer. But as part of her spirited fight for survival she had created her own blog, Cancer-KickinGirl that I followed avidly. I had never met her, but I was really taken by her story, her positive energy and her attitude. During my 52-week streak I tried to dedicate each race to a patient with pancreatic cancer. I knew that I was dedicating this marathon--#32—to Ashley.

Thinking about her spirit buoyed my own. The City of Santa Clarita Marathon is a now-22-year old event. It attracts a total of about 5,000 participants in the full, half, 10K and kid's fun runs. That's not New York, but it's hardly some fly-by-night operation.

By the time we got off the plane, I was still tired but I had mentally adjusted to what I anticipated was going to be a very, very different race experience than the five boroughs of New York.

We hopped into David's car in long term parking and drove directly up to the race expo. One thing Santa Clarita has in common with New York: They're both cities, although Santa Clarita is actually composed of four distinct unincorporated communities: Canyon Country, Newhall, Saugus and Valencia.

The race expo was in the Westfield Town Center, a cool little mall in downtown Valencia. When I walked in the main lobby where the registration tables were set up, I was greeted by a gaggle of TV crews.

"Julie, you just flew across the country and flew back in two days to keep your marathon streak going. How do you feel?"

"I feel like I just went through a washing machine," I said.

"Did you think the decision to cancel the New York City Marathon was a correct one?"

A moot point now, so I sidestepped the question. I talked about what we'd seen in the city, and expressed my hope they'd be able to get everything back to normal as soon as possible.

After that, I spent the afternoon on social media, napping and praying. Yes, I really did. I prayed that I'd be able to finish the race tomorrow. Normally that's not something I worried about. But this had hardly been a normal week.

On my blog, I had made a big deal about how I went from running a marathon with 50,000 to one with 500, which was about how many were opting to run the full 26.2-mile distance in the Santa Clarita event. But as we ran along the next morning, I began to realize that a quiet race in the bucolic northern reaches of Los Angeles County has its advantages. Instead of the concrete of the Big Apple's streets, most of the Santa Clarita Marathon was held on the paseos—that's the Spanish word for trails, and the city has over 20 miles of them designated for the use of pedestrians, runners and bikers. Their trail system includes bridges and tunnels that flow seamlessly over, around or under the roads. "So you never have to deal with cars," Patrick explained.

Besides being kinder to my legs, running along the dirt-packed paseos also allowed me to get into a comfortable rhythm. I relaxed and enjoyed the scenery—the San Gabriel Mountains in the distance, the chaparral-covered hillsides.

I was back in California, and there was something to be said for that.

It was a hot day, and given the tumult of the past few days, I was in no mood to press the pace, so I ran easily, enjoying the scenery and the sweet Santa Clarita air (the mountains block the L.A. smog from drifting into the valley up here.)

It turned out to be a wonderful 28-mile run.

Yes, I managed to actually run two miles further than marathon distance that day.

The reason was a runner named Marjorie. I vaguely knew her from other local races. She was a strong runner and she was well ahead of me for much of the race. But at one point of the course, I saw her. She had dropped back and seemed to be struggling. "I'm going to quit," she declared. I was startled that she even spoke to me. "Okay," was all the response I could think of.

I continued running. After about a mile, I said to myself, "what are you doing? You should never tell anyone to quit." I knew this woman was a quality runner, and maybe I was intimidated by her. But everyone needs encouragement in a marathon, and I felt like I'd failed to give her any. I decided to do something you're not supposed to do in a marathon or any race.

I turned around and ran back. As I did, I reached into my arsenal of shopworn motivational marathon clichés, prepared to bombard her with these.

"You can do it...you got this...you're looking good."

Meanwhile spectators and runners behind me were aghast to see someone going in the opposite direction. "You're going the wrong way!" a few called to me.

"Thanks," I responded wearily. "I know."

I ran for about 10-15 minutes. I couldn't find any sign of Marjorie. She'd probably dropped out shortly after I'd seen her. Counting the time to get back where I'd turned around originally, I estimated that I covered about two extra miles.

Maybe it was just as well. Who knows how she would have

responded to my hackneyed motivational bromides? On the other hand, I imagined the series of emotions she would go through after stepping off the course. First, relief, then anger, then some self-loathing and incrimination. While I'm sure she wasn't psychologically scarred for life, I wondered if she'd ever muster the courage to try this again. And I wondered if she had quit the marathon, whether she was prone to quitting when things got tough in other aspects of life. I thought about how I had gone through some of the same stages in my own life as a marathoner.

Enough being an amateur psychologist—especially coming from me, someone that I'm sure is regarded as a certifiable nut by most of the people she meets, especially during my 52-marathon streak!

I certainly didn't feel crazy that day. Thinking of my dad, New York, and of Ashley (who sadly would lose her battle to pancreatic cancer the next year) gave me renewed focus and drive. By the end of the Santa Clarita Marathon, I knew exactly why I was there—even if the "there" was not where I'd originally expected to be on Nov. 4, 2012.

As I crossed the finish line of my 28-mile marathon, Patrick, the race director, gave me a nice shout-out. "Here comes the Marathon Goddess Julie Weiss from Santa Monica via New York," he said over the PA system. "She's running 52 marathons in 52 weeks to fight pancreatic cancer."

The spectators at the finish line—all of about 50 of them—cheered. I also posed for a fun finish line photo of me surrounded by the cute cheerleading squad of the Canyon High School Cowboys, pompoms and all. Their school motto is: "It's a great day to be a Cowboy!"

And for Cowgirls, too. It was indeed a great day to finish marathon number 32, in the heart of the Santa Clarita Valley.

After the race, I was interviewed by CBS who tracked me from NYC to Santa Clarita; I gave a hug to Pat, who had been so gracious about letting me in the race last minute. David and I walked back to our hotel and came across a public fountain in the Westfield Town Center. It called to me. I sat down, took off my purple Asics and plunked my feet in the water.

"Ah, this feels amazing," I said, as David recorded the moment on his phone. "This will save my feet for the next marathon. Oh wait, I'm not supposed to do this?"

Okay, I'm sorry I stuck my sweaty feet in a public fountain. No one drank out of this water, anyway. But those feet had travelled a long distance over the previous days. I'd gone across the country and back twice, run a marathon on both coasts, and managed to keep the streak going despite being caught up in an epic marathon controversy and brushed by the after-effects of one of the most devastating storms in New York's history. "If I can survive all that," I thought, "I know I can keep going all the way to 52."

As there were still 20 marathons to go, perhaps I shouldn't have been so certain. My confidence, my resolve, my heart, and yes, my soles, would all be tested again in the weeks and months to come.

Chapter 15
How Do You Run a Marathon a Week, Anyway?

People often asked me how much running I did during the weeks I was in pursuit of my 52-marathon goal. The answer: I didn't. Running a marathon every weekend, I had learned, is all about recovery on the weekdays. You're not out on the track trying to get faster, you're not out doing hill repeats in mid-week, as you might be if you were training for one goal race. For me, six or seven days between marathons were about resting and recuperating sufficiently to keep the body whole and muster the energy to go back and run 26.2 miles again...and again...and again.

Here, I was lucky. The post-marathon soreness that many people feel for days, and in some cases weeks after a marathon, didn't affect me too badly. I'd try to walk and stretch as much as possible after the race—starting in the airport. By mid-week, I'd be feeling good.

While I didn't do much running, I did do some strength training every Tuesday. And I had bodywork done every Wednesday, by a sports doc who specialized in myofascial release—a manual therapy technique that focuses on the membranes that wrap and connect our muscles. It's a manual technique, meaning that you lay on a table like a massage as the therapist works on you. But unlike a relaxing massage at a day spa, this is very deep and sometimes painful. However, it seems to work for lots of people, including me. I always felt better the day after one of those treatments.

Friday was travel day—which generally meant, panic day.

With the New York debacle far behind me, another California marathon the next week, and Maui the week after, I felt hopeful. I was inching my way closer, back on my grind, and felt a newfound strength. Plus, donations were coming in strong. I decided to double down on getting the word out via local news channels—it was a grassroots strategy to get the cause on people's minds. Every time I spoke to a reporter, they asked me how I did it. How did I run a marathon per week, and how did I expect to make it through 52 in a year without getting hurt? It was a good question. I gave much of the credit to David who, when he originally planned out my schedule for this year-long undertaking, had recommended that 26.2 would be my weekly running mileage. I would not really train—I just needed to maintain. That could be done by running a race each week.

I still wanted to feel prepared. When we sat down with my Outlook calendar and list of races, we knew we were entering un-chartered territory. I sat on my overstuffed couch with my legs curled under me, and David sat on the chair across from me, pour-ing over the papers.

"I've never gone into a race without running at least some-times beforehand," I told him.

He nodded, understanding.

"Right, right," he said. "But at this volume, you don't re-ally want to put any more pressure on your legs and joints than you absolutely have to."

He thought some more.

"If you really want to, we could get you one of those aqua jogging belts," he said, more asking then telling me. I knew what he was talking about.

"Oh man," I said. "They're pretty dorky."

It's basically a flotation device you wear around your waist so you can run with your head above water and without touching the bottom of the pool. It allows you to work the same muscles you would while running and maintain your aerobic capacity without putting any strain on your body. I thought it might be good to give it a try.

He told me then, that each race should be slower than the last. This would make my recovery time faster. If I went nice and easy, my muscles wouldn't break down as much, and this would be especially important as we got deeper into the schedule. Then, the real kicker. My average marathon time was 3:50. David wanted me to slow it down so that across all 52 races, my average would be 5:30.

"Well, but..." I started. He knew me and was already defending the statement before I could finish my objection.

"It's to keep you healthy, to get you to the finish of every race."

"But even if I'm not getting faster, I don't want to get slower."

"You won't be getting slower, you'll just be running slower. Think about it as taking control of your speed."

I let it go, sighed heavily. I ordered an aqua jogger belt and vowed to try it as soon as it arrived.

It's a clumsy thing, hugging the tender part of your waist, and strapping with a buckle across the flat of your stomach. But it kept me afloat, bobbing up and down like a buoy in the deep end of the pool. Running in the water felt pointless. I didn't move. I just stared at a blank wall and moved my limbs in an awkward jog. I did it for 60 minutes and emerged pruned and cold.

At home, I asked David how many miles I probably ran.

"None," he said. "You just floated in place."

Not funny.

After the first week of aqua-jogging, I dropped that idea. Spending an hour in the pool while working full-time just wasn't going to do it. David said that was fine because rest was more important than running in water.

But he did start calculating all the fuel I put into my body. He advised me to eat more minerals to keep my brain functioning properly. He took my weight at the start of the adventure to figure out how much protein I needed: 70 grams per day. I had to figure out how to squeeze that in. I'm a vegetarian, which makes getting protein a challenge. We bought a slew of vegetarian protein powders and tested them all. I hated most of them, but they became my best go-to snack.

I was hungry all the time. I needed carbs to sustain me and to keep my energy levels up. David and I made a pasta dish—and prepared enough of it on Monday to last us the whole week. We took tortellini, or any kind of pasta we had on hand, and mixed it together with a bunch of vegetables. Even though I would eventually grow tired of eating the same damn pasta mixture every night, it was a miracle food. It kept me going.

Sleep, of course, was necessary. Eight hours was the mark I was supposed to hit, but I'm just not that good at resting. If I wasn't tossing and turning before race weekend, I was on social media connecting with potential donors, survivors, or people struggling with pancreatic cancer. With so much work to do and such a battle to fight, how was I supposed to sleep at night? David would urge me to bed, then annoyingly pass out on the couch next to me while I tried to wrap up text conversations.

The rest of the plan was stretching, foam rolling, getting treatment to work the knots worked out of my muscles. I stretched in the airport, on the plane, in the shower immediately after the race. I took 15 minutes to stretch no matter what. The more I lengthened and strengthened my muscles, the better I felt going into the week.

I wore compression everywhere. Tights, calf sleeves, arm sleeves, tops—wearing these garments was supposed to increase oxygen flow to muscles by 40 percent. Early on, a vendor gave me a pair of pink sparkly knee-high compression socks to run in, and I wore them every race.

During each race, I ate some of David's mystery mineral pills. These were just electrolytes in capsule form. Generally, I took them every 30 minutes, but on warmer days would require a pill approximately every 20 minutes. This prevented me from sodium depletion. Studies have shown, approximately one out of every five marathon finishers are in some degree of hyponatremia. Essentially, they are sodium depleted, which means their bodies can no longer absorb water efficiently. This can become a life-threatening issue. Unlike most that are told to avoid salt, runners need sodium. Other minerals, such as potassium are also critical for proper muscle function. A little calcium, magnesium and others are a bonus as well.

Chapter 16
Running Through Hell in Paradise

The clear sky, fresh air, beautiful flowers, everything at the Honolulu Marathon was perfect, except for me.

Trouble started the night before, when we checked in and realized our room had two separate beds. On any normal trip, this wouldn't have affected me the way it did, but David and I were drifting apart. This bed situation seemed to symbolize exactly what was going on in this relationship.

I could feel his frustration with me growing; the air around us felt heavy. I was annoyed when he was talking, planning, puttering around the apartment talking about the upcoming races. I told him he made me nervous. When he talked about his race group, or track practice, I groaned. Running consumed our weekends, I wanted to keep my weekdays free from hearing about it. I grew furious over the smallest things: dishes left on the counter, a trace of shaving cream in the sink. "David," I'd yell. "I have enough to deal with right now." There was space between us—a space as big as the gap between these two beds in Hawaii.

I complained to him and called down to the front desk to ask for a king bed. But they were booked solid.

"It's fine, Julie," David was speaking in the annoying voice he uses to calm people down.

"David, God, just let me be upset."

We settled into our separate beds and went to sleep.

The alarm went off at 3:45 a.m. I woke up slowly and dragged myself to my suitcase. I searched for my shorts and purple sports bra. I needed my socks and compression sleeves. I started digging, frantically. I couldn't find anything.

"David?"

He was still in bed.

I needed him, I thought I did anyway.

"David," I said, loud. "Are you ever going to get up?"

He stirred. I grumbled. He tossed the Hawaiian floral comforter on the floor and marched to the bathroom. He went in, slammed the door. I froze. I couldn't get dressed. What should I do?

I figured he would calm himself down and say he was sorry when he emerged. But instead, he was fuming.

"You know, Julie, you don't need my help to get dressed," he yelled. "Every single weekend, every single day, is about you. It's about you and I love you and this mission you're on, but give me a break?"

"What are you talking about?" I could feel my voice get stuck in my throat. I knew exactly what he was talking about. I took him for granted all the time. But I needed him, didn't he see that? I just had to get through the next few races, and then we could start over. I would be the girlfriend he wanted me to be. The romance was still there, it was just blocked by the 52.

"You're being selfish," he said. "This is supposed to be bigger than you, but you're really making it all about you. Especially when it comes to me."

"You're being dramatic," I said. "And you're bringing all this up at 4 in the morning? An hour before a race."

He held out his hands and shrugged. "I can't take it anymore, Julie."

He left the room.

"Where are you going?"

I stood in shock, in the middle of this two-bed room. "Dammit." I sat on the floor. I opened my phone and wrote out my dedication to the man I was running for, Curt Wada. I didn't want to run, but this race was for him. I pulled on my compression socks, and I cried.

David came back to the room and walked with me to the start of the race. The silence was bitter and when he took out his camera to film me taking off, I told him to turn it off. I was not feeling any positive energy, and I didn't want any documentation of just how bad this morning was.

Overhead, flashes of light rained down over the runners at the start. I kept my eyes ahead but heard the loud blasts of fireworks. The cheering around me sounded muffled. My eyes watered uncontrollably. "Just get me through," I said a quiet prayer. It was to my Dad, and to Curt.

I dedicated this race to Curt, a beautiful man who worked as a Stage Manager at House of Blues in Anaheim, CA. Music was his passion, especially rock. I made a playlist just for him so we could jam out together as we ran.

Curt's sister Julia contacted me a few weeks before the race to tell me about him. He was diagnosed with pancreatic cancer in

December 2008, and he died two weeks later. His cancer was not treatable, but he underwent chemo for palliative care. Curt was a big guy with a huge presence. He acted as Julia's protector. As an uncle to Julia's son, he babysat all the time and taught him how to ride a bike and play drums. His long hair, the music, his California roots, I felt connected to him. I knew that life and that era. Curt made the best of his wild streak—turned his love of rock n' roll into a career. To see him waste away at such an incomprehensible speed caused extreme trauma to Julia and her family. On Jan. 7, 2009, Curt passed peacefully with his family by his side. His last words to his sister were "Don't worry, I'm okay." They grieved every day. I hoped to ease just some of that pain.

At this point, I wasn't just running races for people who were battling cancer, but for people who were lost, whose family members wanted their memory to live on. Now, I needed Curt as much as his family needed me. I turned my music up loud and started to walk. My limbs wouldn't break into a run, and I accepted that. I just needed to move. I couldn't smile, couldn't cheer. I left my spirit on the hotel room floor.

I knew that in any distance event, a dark thought may come up for a split second. "Just quit," it might say. At mile 13 of the Honolulu Marathon, that thought kept repeating, growing louder. I thought about walking off the course. Quitting. After a few dreary steps, I heard a loud voice yelling, "NO WAY." I looked around. I saw only other runners, deep into their races. Who would have yelled that to me, at that precise moment, as if they were reading my mind? A named popped into my head: Could it be? Curt? Whoever or whatever it was elicited a response. I continued running.

Another great personality picked me up at mile 23. I remembered then words from Bart Yasso, who told me that when you're running marathons in Hawaii, no matter how bad you feel during the race, when you finish, you're in paradise. I wanted to make it to the end to tell David that. I hoped that he could then tell me his frustrations honestly and openly. And that I could tell him in all candor that even when I was being spoiled, the right time and place to start a fight was not the hour before a marathon.

With New York being canceled, the race was huge, well over 25,000 people. I smiled at the runners around me in the homestretch, but after hearing a voice from beyond the grave, not to mention an absent but dear friend, I couldn't help but remain in my own head. There was no whooping or dancing this time. When I got to the end and found David, I wanted to tell him how I felt, but nothing came out. He didn't say much either.

Chapter 17
Three Marathons
in Three Days

"This is the weirdest marathon I've ever run," I whispered to the members of my crew as I came to the fifth mile of the Lake Tahoe Triple Marathon. Three marathons, three days. I was only on day one, and already feeling beat.

David was with me, manning the camera. I brought two other friends, neighbors from Santa Monica, Camille and Aiden, to support me throughout the miles. I figured I'd need three people to complete three marathons.

"Why is it weird?" Camille said. She and Aiden leaned in to hear my thoughts. They held bottles filled with orange liquid, something that looked like juice from the heavens.

"What's that?" I pointed at their drinks.

"Orange juice, squeezed minutes ago." She gave me some to try.

"That's amazing,"

The night before, David and I had rolled into Lake Tahoe—an eight-hour trip from L.A. As usual, we were running behind, speeding to get away on a Thursday. We hurried as much as we could, heading north to the woods. We needed to make it to the expo in time to pick up my bib, but I knew we probably weren't going to make it.

I hoped that the folks manning the expo would take pity on me, understand the long trip we had, and the number of races I was doing. It was impossible to make it to everything on time. When we arrived, just after the 6 p.m. pickup time, I flew through the doors of the Taphouse Grill, looking for anyone associated with the race. An older man was packing things up. I ran up to him.

"I am so sorry, I just got into town, I still need to pick up my bib."

He smirked.

"You're late," he said.

"I know. I had an eight-hour drive out of L.A."

"You could've left earlier."

I couldn't believe it. Who was this guy?

"I'm sorry," I said, more assertive than apologetic. "I'm Julie Weiss, it's nice to meet you."

"I'm the race director," he said. "You know, I don't have to give you the bib tonight. I will, but you could've gotten it tomorrow morning."

I stood there. I needed these three marathons. After the third, I would be halfway through the 52. I wanted to tell him that he was being an ass, but instead I felt myself grow warm and shaky. My eyes—they were tearing. Oh yes, he made me cry.

He handed me my bib.

"See you at 6 a.m. sharp," he said. I felt like I had just been grounded. I met David outside and we went across the street to check into our hotel.

"What happened?" David asked. "You're so upset."

"I think I just got in trouble for being late." I didn't want to explain it much more.

I coached myself down from a meltdown. I tried to understand, to see it from the director's perspective. He needed to prepare for a three-day long event, the logistics of which were likely a nightmare. But I was just a marathoner looking for her bib. I didn't think something so small could make me feel so small, but it did.

I fell asleep in tears.

Rounding the first corner and seeing all three of my support crew members standing in the road with glorious, cold orange juice, I was thankful and tried to put any discomfort or hurt feelings out of my mind.

Here's how the Tahoe Triple works. You start at Lakeside Beach in Lake Tahoe, California and head up to Incline Village in Nevada. Then you stop for the day and show up to the same place you finished the next morning. The second marathon starts just south of Incline Beach, then heads back into California. On Sunday Funday, you start from the point you stopped on Saturday and return to the very place you started. It's one giant loop around Lake Tahoe. The race only allows about 150 participants; more runners can run the individual races, but it's still a small field. There is no crowd support, just tall trees and sweeping views of the lake. It's absolutely stunning, but also at altitude, and a total beatdown on your body.

Day 1: 9/28/2012

At the start of day one, with the tears behind me, I arrived at the line with three layers on. The air was crisp, but the sun was already coming up and beating down.

"It's gonna get warm, fast," David said. I took off my pants, handed them to him. He crumpled them in his hand with Thing. I had tried to get rid of Thing, but I think David kept bringing him back to life.

I kept my sweatshirt and waited at the back of the pack. The man who admonished me the night before now walked across the line, in front of the crowd, carrying an enormous rifle. Oh no, I thought. Here it is, he's going to shoot me for being late.

But no, it was a true shotgun start. He hollered at us to move to the side of the road and BANG! We took off, having to immediately move to the right side of the road to avoid oncoming traffic. The race was small enough that they didn't need to close roads completely, and they depended on runners to know where they were going and stay safe. I could follow a course map now with ease, and I thought that as long as I stayed along the lake, I'd figure it out. I took a deep breath and cruised through the first few miles. The thin mountain air greeted me, and I watched the water out of the corner of my eye, vowing to jump in once this first marathon was over.

David was, of course, right. The sun lifted over the tall pines and it was hot in an instant. I slowed down, taking my pace way down, run-walking at times to even before the fifth mile.

When I finally met my crew and saw the magical orange juice, I was beat. My body temperature was elevated, and all I wanted was to down the orange juice. I felt like it might be the only thing that could save me. And, unlike some races, where every water stop was a multi-course buffet, Tahoe only had the essentials. Water and Gatorade.

"So why is this a weird marathon?" Camille broke me out of my orange juice trance. Her blonde ponytail blew in the wind and she looked flawless. My sweat dripped down my arms and my hair clung to my back. Aiden stood there, waiting to hear my review. Then he explained to me how the orange juice was made right in front of them. I wasn't comprehending. I nodded.

I wasn't sure if they'd ever crewed a race before or knew what to do. They offered orange juice, and that was great at mile five. But I hoped they'd have my cold water, a wet towel, all the stuff I'd packed in a backpack and left with them as the race went on. Where was that backpack, anyway?

"It's just, you're up against traffic. You have to wait for stop lights, and I hardly see other runners. And I keep reminding myself that I have to do this three times this weekend."

"Stay here, stay now, girl," she said. I knew what she meant. I needed to focus on the mile I was in, not in the 60-plus miles ahead.

I continued on, feeling like a slug, hopeful that my crew would bring me another treat the next time I saw them. I fell off my pace even more, staying just ahead of the six-hour cut-off. I knew I could do it, I just had to do so at my own speed. In the heat, I craved water, cold water. I needed something to wash down my trusty mineral pills, but I soon realized that I was apparently too slow for the aid stations to wait for me. I'd turn the bend and see a graveyard of cups, but the tables were folded. I'd missed the only hydration for miles.

I tried not to panic. I knew David and crew would meet me somewhere. The miles ticked by, and I wondered where they were. I needed more sugar, something other than what I was carrying in my pack. I wanted a cold drink and some company. Around the 17th mile, I found them. My crew, sitting at a nice restaurant.

"Is that a goddess?" They cheered, looking up from their turkey and brie sandwiches.

I rolled my eyes, asked for water. Just a few more miles to go.

"How's lunch?" I said.

I didn't have enough energy to tell them that the aid stations were gone, that I was out there practically by myself, low on my own lukewarm water, and craving all the fresh-squeezed orange juice in the world. I wanted to scream, where are my race-day go-to necessities? Instead, I left them with their sandwiches. Food was making me queasy.

I had to let it go. Seven miles and I could jump in the lake.

Day 2: 9/29/2012

Daybreak on Saturday and I would rather dive into the lake with cement blocks on my feet than be out on the road. My legs felt like cement anyway, so what difference would it make. The lack of hydration and heat I experienced the day before had depleted my entire system. Six miles in, my crew is there, cheering me on. I stop and walk. It was going to be a long day out along the lake.

"How do you feel?" Camille asked me and adjusted my bib for me. I was thankful for her then, she was there when I needed her most. All was forgiven.

"I feel like I'm going to cry," I said.

"How do you feel, physically?"

"I feel pretty good," I lied. What else was I going to do? Complaining wouldn't get me any closer to my goal. "My legs are hanging in there, and I'm going downhill now."

The course wound around mountainous roads, up and

down, cutting in and out of traffic. At mile 13, I asked for an energy drink: Redline. With 360mg of caffeine per eight-ounce bottle, I
knew that could wake me up. I pounded the triple berry flavor and
felt the back of my neck tingle.

"Woo," I let out a quiet yell. Like jet fuel, that stuff coursed
through my veins and sent me off, running—really running. "I'm
close," I repeated over and over, seeing the big trees and mile signs
fly by. I wasn't actually breaking speed barriers, but it felt fast and
effortless.

The stopping point that day was on a busy street with traffic at my back. I made my way down a bike lane and crossed the
cone barrier with my arms up in the Goddess pose. "Two down!" I
shouted. "More like 25 down. Tomorrow I'll be halfway!"

Another race down, another lake swim, and shockingly, a
full night's sleep.

Day 3: 9/30/2012

For race three, slow runners could start whenever they
wanted to, as long as it was before 8:00 a.m. It was Sunday-Funday,
which meant a low-pressure atmosphere with plenty of walkers as
well as runners along the course. This time, the roads weren't as

full, and we ran past beautiful bays with the most sweeping views of the course.

I felt better. With two marathons behind me, and a ton of tears let loose in Nevada, I was ready to end the three days of torture. My body seemed to be ready to get it done, and my legs took off from the start in a fierce rhythmic cadence.

Even though I felt better, I knew I was beat. My face felt puffy, my eyes sunk in, and my mind—well I wasn't forming perfect sentences, even in my head.

This is where the mind shuts down and lets the body do its thing. I'd experienced flow—the state where your body just takes over and your mind is quiet and you don't even feel like you're working—a few times in races. This was one of them. My memory of the third and final race of the Tahoe Triple is mostly blank—a beautiful white space after two days of pain.

I will not forget, however, what occurred at the finish. A woman in yellow approached me.

"Hi there," she said.

"Hi! Did you finish too?"

"Oh yes, I did."

She didn't look any worse for the wear.

"Congratulations."

"You're Julie Weiss, Marathon Goddess?"

I nodded. It was fun to be recognized, even when I felt like I was delirious.

"My friend asked me to find you at this race," she said. "She's following you. Her husband died last year. I'm in town from South Carolina, running here, and I told her that if I found you, I would get an autograph."

I was floored. I never thought I would ever give an autograph, but more so, that I was making a difference in someone's life all the way across the country.

"She called me yesterday to ask if I had found you yet," she went on.

The tears started up again. She handed me a shirt and a magic marker. "Will you sign it for her?"

"Oh my gosh, yes," I wiped my face quickly. I wanted so badly to meet the woman in South Carolina and give her a hug. Instead, I spent too long scrawling a message out on her shirt, something that was likely incomprehensible and looked like a 5-year-old wrote it. I apologized for my handwriting.

"Oh honey," the woman said, "you just ran three marathons. I think you're forgiven."

Her kindness made my day. I grabbed her and hugged her.

I promised that on my next big tour of marathons, I would run one in South Carolina.

"We do have some that aren't too hot," she said, with a chuckle. I wasn't sure I believed her.

My crew started gathering my things. The race announcer allowed me to give a little stump speech and celebrated my half-way mark with me. I told the crowd who I was running the race for and that nothing was going to stop me. Even with a rocky start, the Tahoe Triple ended up being one of my favorite races. It was a little off-beat, but man, it brought out the best in me.

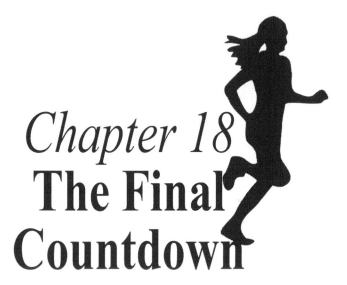

Chapter 18
The Final Countdown

With just ten more marathons to go, I boarded the Delta flight to Mississippi. This race, the Mississippi Blues Marathon in Jackson, would be my 42nd. What a wild thing, I thought to myself as we took off from LAX, to have run 41 marathons. I laughed, thinking of how hard it once was to run from one lifeguard stand to another. I could almost hear my dad laugh too, if I listened hard enough. I hoped he remembered me trying to hold a plank in front of him. Now look at what I'm doing, Dad.

I made it to my hotel room by midnight. The woman at the front desk of my hotel offered to give me a ride to the start line.

Her beautiful, buttery twang seemed contagious. I wanted to call everyone "sugar" or "honey." I fell under the southern spell almost instantly.

Races by this point started blurring together. Faces I saw, I thought I'd recognized from the last weekend. Mile markers, too—race starts, courses, aid stations, expos. In the moment, I loved them all. After the race, I couldn't quite piece it all together. Was it the Hoover Dam Marathon where I saw that really tan guy with the mullet? Or was that at the California International Marathon? Oh, and that looks like that guy who tripped over his shoes at the start of the Route 66 race. I helped him up, does he recognize me? I don't think so. Is that the lady who sang the Canadian National Anthem at the Toronto Waterfront Marathon? Can't remember.

David was unable to make it to many of the races now. We'd both used vacation days, and it was expensive to fly two people all around the country. Plus, I could tell he was still bitter about the little quarrels we kept getting into. And no matter how many times we talked it out, and I apologized, hurt feelings remained. I thought of him back at home, coaching happy runners who were grateful for his guidance. I missed him.

I thought of him, and then of all the people who had my

back. Throughout my 52-week challenge, I saw people I knew from home or Facebook or Twitter.

There were more and more of these kind souls: Posts and emails from folks looking to get races dedicated to them or loved ones were now pouring in. I was writing posts for three or four people at a time. Honored as I was, it was incredibly sad to hear about their struggles and know that so many people were affected by this disease. After a while, it felt like I was reading their stories in my dreams. What had started with one man, Maurice Weiss, and the struggles we had, the pain in his last months, and my continuing self-discovery, had grown in a way that I could have never predicted. I hoped I was helping the cause, but the more requests for dedications I received, the more victims or survivors I met, the more perplexed I was why, with so many victims of this terrible disease, it was still the most underfunded form of cancer in terms of donations and research dollars?

Something else strange was happening: Marathons had been getting easier. I wasn't sore at all. I was flying through races, and it was getting more enjoyable. It felt almost magical. Like I had the energy from all of these people I was running for helping me. I didn't want it to end.

I couldn't believe it when I woke up in my own bed on St.

Patrick's Day 2013. The day was finally here—I would be running my last marathon of the year; my goal was just 26.2 miles away. I was lucky to have the L.A. running community rallying around me, along with local press and the 15,000 people who were supporting my effort online. Because I'd made it so far, because there was almost no denying that I would make it, the national media took notice. NBC wanted to do an interview before the race. Reporters from various newspapers would catch me along the course. I reminded myself over and over to mention my website and tell people where they could donate.

I jumped out of bed.

"Good morning!" David said, cheerfully. Despite the distance that had grown between us, we put it aside that day.

"Good morning!" I replied warmly.

It was still dark. I was used to that. I flipped on all the lights in the apartment and grabbed my smoothie.

"This is it," I looked at David and furrowed my brow. "Can you believe it?"

"Of course, I can!" His joy spread to me. I laughed out loud, a big hearty laugh that caught in the back of my throat.

"We're gonna do it, David," I yelled.

"I know!"

I felt the way I had before the Rome Marathon, one year earlier, and man how I missed that feeling of anticipation. I'd spent the past 12 months just getting to the next phase, promising myself it would get easier.

And near the end, it had. Now, about to finish, all the exhaustion vanished. I knew it was pure adrenaline coursing through my body, but I figured there was enough there to carry me through the entire race.

I grabbed my purple sports bra, my black shorts, my fuel belt, the Hawaiian purple flower for my hair. I brushed my mane back into a ponytail. I wondered if I should start with a sweatshirt. I opened the window. My special arm sleeves would do.

Next, I pulled on my 12th pair of Asics GT-1000's, which felt like a security blanket. I'd already worn through 11 pairs. I grabbed my backpack full of postrace gear and snacks.

I turned to David. He was going to run with me—the first time since Marathon 33. He had his purple tee-shirt, a pair of shorts, and he was ready. That was all he needed. I hugged him hard.

"Oh my God," I said.

He laughed.

Laurence Cohen, the former public relations director for the L.A. Marathon, pulled up in his silver Buick Regal, accompanied by a CNN cameraman, who would be filming me. I kissed David goodbye. As he had to pick up some of the runners from his group, he was driving separately.

I wanted to make a caustic crack to Laurence about David's car, parked nearby. "Think there's a homeless person living in that trunk?"

But I didn't. Making fun of David and his sorry vehicle that morning would have taken away from the joy of the moment—and I wanted us to think of this glowing time, the hour before the biggest race of my life, and just remember how pure and magical it was.

This race, I would dedicate every mile to a different person. Those special arm sleeves I mentioned? I had written their names on them. Some had sent messages to me, and I kept their words in my heart, and dutifully inscribed them on my sleeves:

Mile 1: Judith Maiman

Mile 2: John Sam Chee

Mile 3: David G. Hollander

Mile 4: Edmund C Bechtold

Mile 5: Doug and Jeff Brand, brothers taken from this horrible disease less than a year apart

Mile 6: Spyros Sipsas

Mile 7: K. Bradbury & Curt Sandoval

Mile 8: Robert Holloway

Mile 9: Ron Smith

Mile 10: Patrick Powers

Mile 11: Grandma Gerry

Mile 12: John Price

Mile 13: Buck

Mile 14: Nancy Kramer

Mile 15: For my sweet fiancé Edward J. Demyan who would have turned 50 this week; March 15, 2013. Missing you every day EJD–this week is especially hard. -M. Mackulin

Mile 16: Adam Zauder

Mile 17: Amo Cappelli

Mile 18: Herman C. Atienza

Mile 19: Noel Irvine

Mile 20: Please dedicate mile 20 to my father, Rodney Buffington, who also lost his battle to pancreatic cancer after just 20 short weeks! -A. Winkle

Mile 21: Lora Gudbranson

Mile 22: Yitzchak ben Chaim Zelig

Mile 23: Paul Perkovic & Team Molli- Strongest woman I know!

Mile 24: Francis P. Urban

Mile 25: Ron Bowker

Mile 26.2: In memory of Melissa Miller and her heroic five-year battle with pancreatic cancer

At the start line, I was surrounded by a sea of purple. People who knew it was my 52nd and wanted to run—some survivors, others with family members they were dedicating races to—joined me at the start, all in purple tees. Members of the Pancreatic Cancer Action Network were there. I held two purple balloons. The sun started to shine, and I felt a wave of joy, and with an electric feeling in the air, we started. This was the culminating moment—the race I was waiting for. I just wanted to move, but at the same time, I didn't want the journey to end.

My friend Mark from my running group made purple shirts that said Team Julie, with a picture of me and the words "52 marathons in 52 weeks" on the other side. About 20 of my friends surrounded me in these shirts as I ran.

Over the loudspeaker, they called my name as I ran through the starting arch.

"There she is," the announcer yelled, "Julie Weiss. Fifty-two in 52!"

Screams surrounded me, cheers, and chants. Steve Mackel

of Sole Runners would be running the marathon with me, filming the whole thing for his Marathon.TV webcast. I don't think he was ready for the amount of cheering I was going to do, for the whole race. He asked how I was doing.

"This feels surreal," I said. "But now that I'm running, I'm good, I'm free!"

I celebrated the diversity of my city that day, which unfolds through the various neighborhoods along the course. I danced with dragons, and jammed out with a mariachi band, and fist pumped to a drum line. I found my friend Alberto, who runs in bare feet, and who on that day, was completing his 34th. Jenny from Pancreatic Cancer Action Network was out on the course, and when I saw her, I almost cried. I hugged her and rubbed all my sweat on her. I told her she was my family. It was a blur—all of it—all the high fives and bands. I couldn't believe it was my last marathon and how so many people I saw along the course knew me as the Marathon Goddess, running for a cause. I felt truly blessed. I knew that the universe had led me to this moment, that everything in my life got me to this point.

At mile 10, news stations grabbed me for a quick sound bite. Costumed Marathon Man grabbed my waist and gave me a hug. I raised my arms on Hollywood Boulevard, then ran down

Ventura Boulevard, and realized, I only had nine miles to go.

I turned a corner, and there was another familiar face. With long black hair, a black hoody, a black bandana on his forehead, and a mustache. It was Frank.

"This is my ex-husband," I yelled to the entourage that had gathered around me by now. I was probably the only woman in the universe who said those words and felt truly happy to see him standing there. "I can't believe you're here."

"Of course," he said. He held a photo of me from the L.A. Times that he'd cut out and glued to poster board. What a guy. "I told you I'd be here. You look great."

I laughed, thinking back to when he saw me at my first marathon, where I looked like an old lady stumbling along the course. Now I was quite literally dancing my way through the miles.

As I ran past the VA Hospital at mile 21, the hardest, hilliest part of the L.A. course, the feeling started to sink in. It was almost over. I was happy, sad, overwhelmed. I felt unstoppable. I belted, "We've got this" over and over. I ran along spectators, slapping every outstretched hand. Then, with less than 5K to go, a band on the course started singing my name to the tune of the old Wilson Pickett song, "Mustang Sally," with its memorable "ride, Sally, ride" chorus. My group ad-libbed the chorus.

"All she wants to do is run around, Julie; run, Julie, run."

With less than a mile to go, I grabbed my dear friend Lupe, who wore a purple flower in her short, dark hair. Lupe, fighting her own battle, never imagined one day someone would be dedicating the L.A. Marathon to her. She asked if she could cross the finish with me, and I said, absolutely, of course. We finished, side by side. We stood together, smiling so hard my cheeks felt like they might break. David came up behind me, right there for me at the end like he always was.

"Oh, babe," he said.

I grabbed him and held him close.

"We did it!"

I finished in 5:17 with my arms in the air and two purple balloons still in hand. I let one balloon go. That moment was for Maurice, my dad, my cheerleader, and my greatest inspiration.

"We're gonna beat this thing," I screamed. "Let it go!"

I released the other balloon, a symbol to everyone I ran for and would continue to run for.

My year-long odyssey had come to an end. Later we would tally up the numbers:

Fifty-two weeks, 52 marathons.

Two countries, 17 states.

One year, 1,362.4 miles.

279 hours, 39 minutes, and 31 seconds running.

At home, in Santa Monica that afternoon, surrounded by friends, family, fans, and supporters, I couldn't express how grateful I felt. I received calls from news outlets—Natalie Morales from the Today Show wanted to do a story about the marathons.

The day after the race, I felt a crazy nervous energy. I didn't have a race the following week. I didn't have to go anywhere. I paced around my apartment. I knelt down and rubbed Jessie's fluffy face. "Oh Jessie, what should I do with myself?"

I decided I would go for a run. These would be the first miles I'd do without a bib on in more than a year. I told myself I would do five. By the time I looked at my watch, I'd already run eight.

Chapter 19
Depression
and Renewal

I knew all about post-marathon letdown. I'd dealt with it before. You train for 12 weeks, sometimes more, and then you cross the finish line after 26.2 miles and that's it. It's over. All the hard work, all the time spent worrying about your nutrition and shoes and race day gear. The anticipation leading up to that race turns into adrenaline that you burn within the first eight miles. Then you struggle through, make it to then end, and what's next? For everything you do leading up to a marathon, it feels like there should be a parade in your honor. But the reality is, you're just another runner.

Now, I was facing post-marathon letdown 52 times all at once.

I was a different person now. I started the journey as an idealistic and naïve woman—someone who was still finding her way in life and searching for a bigger meaning. Though running gave me the tools to recover from the mess I was before, there was a lot I never knew about myself. I also found the worst version of myself—a tired, pissed-off Julie who took her frustrations out on the people closest to her. There was more, too. I learned that I had more strength inside me than I could ever imagine, and that nothing in life is a coincidence—every person, every encounter, everything you do has a greater purpose.

But what was I supposed to do with all this new knowledge? I thought about David, who was back at home now dozing on the couch. David was there for me every step of the way, and yet, about halfway through, I'd stopped thanking him. I just expected him to be there. When he tried to tell me that he felt neglected or taken advantage of, I acted like I didn't have time to deal with his emotions.

I started my walk back to the car, which was parked just a half-mile away. I plodded along, my legs for the first time in a year feeling robotic and unruly. Just another step, just one more, I told them. I was out of breath by the time I made it.

In the morning, I headed to my office. I settled into my

desk chair, turned on my computer, and checked emails. My colleagues seemed happy enough to have me back on my normal routine; I smiled weakly when they handed me files or asked if I could work on new projects. I agreed with an eager head nod, but inside I felt like screaming. The work I did at my 9-5 wasn't what I felt my purpose in life was. It felt agonizing to have to devote a solid day to something that only paid bills. It was necessary, I knew that, but I also couldn't shake the feeling that my real work was not done.

The worst part was, people I'd connected to throughout the year, members of my Facebook page who have cancer, people whose journeys and battles I've followed, were dying. I watched them go, one by one, throughout my journey and I knew the pattern would continue when I finished the last marathon. But I didn't want to believe it. I wanted my symbolic gesture to literally change the world. But like I'd said so many times before, pancreatic cancer is basically still a death sentence. We are years away from changing that, regardless of how many races we run or dollars we raise.

The whole week that followed the race, I'd been supercharged by my accomplishment and floated through the days ready for a weekend where I could just sleep and cuddle with my dog. But anxious energy filled the air inside my house. I opened all the windows to let it go, tried to get a good rest before the work week, took that slow and painful walk, and nothing. Darkness crept in quickly. And now I sat at my desk, feeling alone and defeated. I looked around at the people I saw every day and felt like no one understood. I knew I was in the office during most of the week, but it felt like I wasn't here for a year. This transition back to normalcy should've been a welcome relief—that's what I had told myself and my colleagues.

Interviews stopped.

The media stopped calling. I knew that if I stopped spreading my message in such a widespread way, the donations would stop. I can be honest, it was a blow to the ego.

How could my highest point lead to such a devastating low? It happened so quickly.

At home, David noticed my mood shift.

"You need a new goal," he said.

"You sound like I didn't just accomplish something major," I shot back.

He sighed. I was looking to fight, trying to pick at him. He wasn't about to bite.

"Julie," he started. I knew he was going to try to logically and rationally explain something to me.

"Save it," I said.

"I'm going to go," he said. Even though we had moved in together at the start of the 52, David kept his condo just down the road. He rarely stayed there, and started making plans to rent it out, but lately, he'd been spending more and more time on his own, away from me.

"You're just going to leave?"

"Yes."

Our relationship had been on the rocks already—the amount of strain we faced during the year prior had made us both question whether it was worth it to keep hanging on to one another. I knew I was wondering if I could spend the rest of my life with a man who drove me crazy with his corny sense of humor and inability to actually fight.

I thought David lacked passion. I told him so. I was so used to relationships that were volatile, explosive. Where love-making and fighting had fire. But David was kind, gentle. He argued by asserting himself. Often, he just kept things to himself and got very quiet when he was very mad.

"This is exactly what I'm talking about when I say it's impossible for us to have a conversation about our differences."

"No, Julie, you mean a conversation about your differences with me."

It stung. I knew what he meant. His biggest problem with me was that I wasn't appreciative of him.

"I'm sorry," I said. I meant it. "It's just, I have this terrible feeling that this whole year wasn't big enough."

 I was letting it all out there.

"Julie, that's crazy," he said. "No one can take away what you accomplished."

"Yeah. But. What do I do now?

"What?"

"It's all over."

"Isn't my attention good enough?"

"Yes, of course, but…"

"You're never satisfied."

David was right. He walked out the apartment door, shutting it softly. I knew I had hurt him, but I told him the truth. All of the feelings I was dealing with didn't have anything to do with him, and perhaps that was part of the problem. While I tried to battle through the 52, and now its aftermath, I'd stopped paying attention to my rock, my greatest supporter. I didn't want to think it, but I was worried. Would I end up losing David, too?

About a month later, it was Marathon Monday, Patriot's Day, and I put a hidden window up on my computer screen at work to watch the Boston Marathon. I remembered running it in the heat a year ago, Dino at my side. Marathon #2. It felt like a decade ago. It was ideal weather for the runners, and I watched the elites take off. The camera crews followed the lead packs, and I smiled as I saw familiar spots along the course.

With the sound on my computer off, I would check in and out throughout the day, with another browser open to check Twitter. I did some work, then checked in. Did some more work, then saw a "Breaking News" banner flash across my screen. Strange. I looked at my open stream of Boston coverage and saw the word: "Bomb."

I unmuted my computer.

"There's a bomb, in Boston," I said it to my coworkers who had gotten the same breaking news message. They came over to look on my screen.

"It was at the marathon, at the finish," one woman said. "Julie, do you know anyone there?"

Yes, I knew people there. My heart started pounding. I texted David: "Are you watching?"

"Yes. Worried."

I called him. Who did we know there? How would we find out if everyone was safe? The images on the screen, the smoke pluming from the finish, the cameras cut away, but I could already see people down in the streets.

We turned on NBC's coverage, with Savanah Guthrie continuing to update the death toll and number of people injured. Just a month ago, she had called herself "wimpy" when she heard about my marathon story. Now she was covering the most tragic news event in running history. I watched in horror as the news helicopters chased the suspects—brothers—around the city. One wore a white hat. They said they were carrying backpacks.

I had so many Road Runners I knew at that race, and all finishing around the 4-hour mark. The time on the clock when the entire race was halted was 4:09:23. In the hours that went by after, I heard from all the people I was worried about. They were safe. But three people were dead. 264 more were injured.

I knew that road races, I knew that the sport and running culture I loved, would never be the same.

The next morning, I woke up, and I did the only thing I knew that would help me heal: I went for a run.

306 | Julie Weiss

Chapter 20
A Grand Proposal

The bombing in Boston snapped me out of my self pity.
I started running like an average, everyday runner again. It was
quite a transition, going from running 26.2 miles once a week, to
logging a few, short runs before work. Did I have a new, big goal
on my agenda? Yes. I had to remind myself that my main goal,
raising $1 million dollars didn't just go away after the 52. There
was no concrete window of time—I was the only person dissatis-
fied with the $230,000 I had handed over to the Pancreatic Cancer
Action Network. And so, I decided that I would make good on my
goal to run another 52 marathons by 2020. I would start almost
right away. I put the San Diego Marathon on the schedule for early
June. It was crazy to consider that a marathon felt like a small goal,

especially considering where I was only five years before.

Though David and I broke up, cancelling our engagement, we still talked nearly every day. My ring finger felt oddly naked without a ring on it, and my life felt empty. It was quiet. Just me and Jessie at home. Friday night dinners with my mom and kids. But no David to greet me when I came home from work. He wasn't there when I wanted to complain about a run, and he wasn't jogging up the stairs to my apartment Saturday afternoons after his run club practice.

David actually went with me to San Diego. There, we attended a *Spirit of the Marathon II* premier the Saturday night before the race. It was weird. We stayed in a room together. We knew we were still not really together, yet it felt almost normal, like we were supposed to be. We looked at each other, and without saying it, I knew what he was thinking. I was thinking it too. What do we do now?

After the race, I missed him. I called him. A lot. And he called me.

"Hey Julie!"

"Hey David."

"What are you doing?"

"Oh, I'm just about to walk down to Starbucks," I paused.

"You want me to bring you a tea?"

"I'm just getting back from a run, and I'm going to shower," he said. "Maybe tomorrow?"

"Yes, I would like that," I said, "You know, I race Kona next week. Remember going to Kona last year?"

"Oh yeah that was a good one," he said.

"I think that is the first place I tried to get Thing to disappear."

He laughed. "I can't wait to hear about your fall season."

"Ha, yeah, I've already got a plan!"

I walked down to Starbucks with Jessie. I loved the slower pace of life now. I'd adjusted to long runs on my home turf and long walks to grab coffee and stare at the high-rise apartments on the Santa Monica coast. Whenever David and I walked along the Santa Monica Pier, I'd tell him about my dream to live right on the shore. I had pictured us living together in one of those complexes, with big windows, and a screen door that we could throw open and let the sea air in. He liked this idea, this dream.

I thought about that dream and I thought about him.

Man, I wasn't over David.

The first time we got engaged had been so sweet in so many ways. I thought maybe I took his romantic side for granted. He told me an amazing story just a few months before the 2011 Chicago Marathon, which we were scheduled to run.

It was the memory of him as a 13-year-old boy, who had come to Chicago with a group of kids from his hometown in Toledo, Ohio. The group was staying at the Drake Hotel, which was once a destination for the very upper-class and A-list celebrities.

After dinner one night, he decided to explore and walked down an old staircase he found. The stairs, he said, felt endless and he walked through old doors only to find more stairs, and against his instincts, he continued to descend. He opened a white door at the bottom of the stairway, and at last there were no more stairs, yet it was completely black. All by himself, in complete darkness, he walked in. A few inches in front of him, from where he stopped, was a low wooden railing. As his eyes adjusted to the low light, he could see below him. And what he saw was magic: An elegant, brilliantly bright red carpet. Above, on the ceiling, there were six enormous chandeliers. It was the Grand Ballroom, of the Drake Hotel. This was the most amazing room David had ever encountered in his entire young life.

He told me he immediately thought of the movie "The King and I." The king, played by Yul Brynner, waltzed across a grand ballroom alone with Debra Kerr in his arms. Then, he imagined himself and the girl of his dreams waltzing all over the football field-sized grand ballroom. In his daydream, he stopped dancing, got down on one knee, opened a box with a ring, and asked her to marry him. *This is it*, he decided then and there. It was his dream to propose to his wife-to-be in that ballroom.

I couldn't imagine that a 13-year-old boy could have a heart like that. After we ran the marathon in Chicago, we were out having celebratory marathon drinks. David asked a friend of ours who knew the city where the Drake was and he told him that the Drake was one block away. It was meant to be. David took me to the Drake. He asked a hotel employee if he could see The Grand Ballroom. When he had originally told me the story about his youthful exploration of the Drake, he didn't mention the name of the hotel or even the city, so I wasn't sure what he was leading me to. The front desk worker told us the ballroom was locked up and out of use, but he said we could check it out if we really wanted to. David nodded eagerly, and we followed along to the supposedly locked door to the grand ballroom, that was actually opened, as if we were expected.

I saw the chandeliers, the red carpet, wide open doors, and a huge dance floor.

"Would you like to dance?" David asked.

"Why of course," I said. He taught me a waltz step and he dragged me around the floor. We both laughed, enjoying the moment, basking in our accomplishment and our love.

After a brief dance, he led me to a chair, and let me sit. Then, he bent down on a knee and asked, "Julie, will you marry me?"

Suddenly I put two and two together. "Is this the place?" I said. I had tears in my eyes.

David nodded.

"Yes," I said. "Oh, my God." I burst out crying with joy.

It was a dream, a beautiful day. Our passion was tangible and our love so pure, it proved stronger than a few quarrels. Maybe, I thought now, four years and one 52-marathon-streak later, all we needed was a break.

###

Not long after that, I met David for lunch at one of the places near Santa Monica Pier. It wasn't awkward at all. We chatted like old friends, which we were.

"So, tell me about your plan," he said.

"Well, I want to run a bunch more races," I said. We both laughed. "But seriously, I want another BQ.

"Really?"

"Yeah!"

"When?"

"L.A. But not this upcoming one, the next one."

"That gives us time."

I wasn't planning to recruit him to help me again, but he started thinking about a training program right away. Talking running was natural for us, and we fell back into our roles easily. He was the coach, and I was the runner. But then I stopped that train of conversation.

"Hey, how are you doing?"

"Julie, we talk nearly every day. I'm great."

"Yeah. Good. I just wanted to ask."

"How's Jessie?"

"She's still the best. Do you want to visit her?"

We walked back to my apartment and grabbed Jessie to go on a walk. She was, of course, excited to see David. We agreed to meet again after Kona. We'd discuss a game plan for my next BQ, and we would text and talk every day until then.

We talked about how the stress of the 52 races had really taken its toll on both of us. We realized that we'd strained our love by submitting it to a crazy adventure. Yet, we were still together, almost all the time. Still friends, and our passion grew stronger every day. At a certain point, we had a whimsical idea: We decided to try to eat at a restaurant on each mile of the L.A. Marathon course. Our love and running, particularly of that race, always coincided. Besides, we're runners, so we are hungry a lot.

"David," I called to him one day in February as I was getting ready to go on a run.

"Yeah babe?"

"You know what would be really cool?"

"Huh?"

"If I BQ'ed in L.A. and if I got proposed to at the finish line."

There was silence.

"See ya later!"

I ran out the door, hoping that was a good enough hint. Even if he didn't do a big marathon proposal, I wanted him to know that I wanted to spend the rest of my life with him.

When I lined up to run the L.A. Marathon on March 15, 2015, I felt BQ-ready.

I ran through the familiar streets and sights of my hometown. Like the song says, I love L.A. A little more than halfway through, I was sure I was going to have the juice to propel me to a 3:50 BQ standard. It was a blistering hot day, and temperatures reached 88 by noon. I got to mile 20 and I felt that all too familiar feeling of hitting the wall. I was crushed. What happened? I trained so hard, 80-mile weeks. How could this be happening, again? At mile 21, the Hirshberg Foundation's Purple People marathon party was in full swing. A huge sea of volunteers and pancreatic cancer survivors were there cheering me. I saw Lupe. I smiled, I knew today was not my BQ day, but seeing her face put all that in perspective. This was way more important. We took a picture and I kept going. As I withered in the heat, my nine-minute miles felt like 12-minute miles. At this point the only thing I could think about was maybe, just maybe David had taken the not-so-subtle hint and would be at the finish line waiting for me with a ring.

As I started to make it to the finish, I saw David pop out from the spectator area. He's here, I thought, but is he really going to propose? My heart was beating so fast now, and it wasn't from the exertion of running. Could this be our moment? How did he even get into the finish line chute with security being so tight? But he was there, just as he was always there for me, from Lake Tahoe to New York; in dark tunnels beneath Seattle and eerie moonlit Nevada landscapes. I heard the announcers call out my name as I crossed the finish line. Now David was behind me and as I turned around, he stopped and got down on one knee on the pavement, that glistened with spilled water and Gatorade.

"Hey," I said.

"Hey, great job," he said. "I have something for you," he said. I was almost in tears. He is really going to do this.

"Julie, will you marry me?"

He held the ring between two fingers—his mother's ring, the one she wore for 53 years of happy marriage.

"Oh!" I squealed. He made it all look so easy; so smooth. Only later what I learn what a production it had been. The security at a big city marathon like L.A. is unrelenting, particularly since the bombings in Boston in 2013. David had dodged security people who didn't know he was a harmless man in love. As they closed in on him, he saw a friend from the running community who was also a race volunteer. She escorted him inside the finish area, and he was relieved, though his palms were sweating, and he couldn't help but think he was going to drop the ring. I was stunned that he managed to make this magical moment a reality.

"Yes!" I screamed. My arms raised over my head for the second time that day, "Yes!"

We were married a little over a month later, on April 24, 2015. David's father was about to celebrate his 90th birthday and invited us to have our wedding that same weekend. We flew out to Toledo to celebrate our nuptials, and my new father-in-law's birthday, with David's family. Everything worked out the way it was supposed to. We both got our dream proposals, and we were with each other, and that was all that really mattered.

Chapter 21
A Marathon Century and Beyond

Later in his life, my father reinvented himself. He went from being the man who wore stiff suits and went to an office every day, to an actor. He won parts in commercials and finally got to channel his performer spirit into profession. But although he did make a major change in his career, I don't think he was ever sad to be confined to a desk job. To him, life was a stage and the people around him were his greatest audience.

Marathons became my stage. Running was where I could break free and literally sing, dance, yell, and zig zag all I wanted. Not many people have completed 52 marathons in 52 weeks, and I plan to keep running more and more. There is nothing stopping me from continuing onward. It's been five years since I ran the 52. I said I would run 52 more marathons by 2020, and I'm well on my way. In 2015, with renewed energy from my marriage to David, I decided to run 14 more marathons and make the following L.A. Marathon my 100th of all time.

Still, I ask myself every day, "What's next?" After David and I got married, we moved into a cozy apartment that overlooks the beach in Santa Monica—just like we always dreamed. I have a wall with all my race medals that I look at every day and add to as often as I can. Jessie is still kicking, even though she's an old girl now. She's really slowed down, and sometimes I carry her outside and plop her on the grass, so she doesn't have to use her energy to make it to the elevator. I reminisce about the runs we used to do together, and I pat her fluffy head and thank her for keeping me going.

When I run on the beach, I ask for inspiration. I continue to dedicate races and raise money. We're up to $500,000 now, running for the Hirshberg Foundation for pancreatic cancer research. I am so grateful for, so blessed to have known people who are willing to help fight this with me.

I also have a quiet goal: I'd still like to qualify for Boston one more time, just to prove I can. It seems pedestrian compared to my other feats, and yet it's what's burning in my heart right now.

Back to that question: I'll never stop asking what's next for me. I will chase goal after goal and continue the rollercoaster of emotions, knowing that I need to enjoy the moments and the process, and even appreciating the grief I feel once one goal is complete, because that's who I am. I am never finished. I will not stop in my fight to end pancreatic cancer, and I will not stop evolving as a wife, mother, grandmother, friend, runner, woman, and daughter.

To me, the greatest lesson I learned was understanding that each and every one of us is a work in progress, incomplete in our quest, but still lightning rods of greatness. Find your light. Keep your light shining. If everyone ignites their passion, think of how bright the world will be.

Chapter 22
Straight Talk For Those Who Want to Kick-Start Their Lives

"Dear Julie: I have been so inspired by your story. I'm considering launching myself into a similarly insane program. :-D What advice would you give to someone looking to do what you have done?"

"Marathon Goddess: Thank you so much for all you've done. In-

spirational does not cover it. Any advice or guidance you can pro-vide would be much appreciated so I can avoid rookie mistakes and learn from your experience."

"Julie: I recently set myself a goal to achieve things in the fight against breast cancer. As I'm completely new to this, I have ab-solutely nowhere to begin. How would I put together, say, 52, half marathons around the world in 52 weeks? Thank you in ad-vance and I await your reply."

These three messages, received over the past year, are fair-ly typical of the hundreds I've gotten, through Facebook or emails on my website, since I completed my 52 in 52 weeks.
I respond individually, but usually with a similar message.

First, I thank them. I'm genuinely touched that they would come to me for advice.

Second, I congratulate them for being interested in doing something that will benefit themselves and others.

Third, I offer this advice to those who are specifically inter-ested in attempting 52 marathons in 52 weeks:

Don't do it.

At least not yet. There's a reason only two or three people, including me, have ever even tried doing so many marathons in such a concentrated period of time. One of them is sanity, or a lack thereof. But the others, seriously, are the enormous time and expense, and the toll it could take on the body. I was lucky. People who meet me often seem surprised that I'm not in a wheelchair.

There are reasons for that, some of them smart training (I thank my husband David for that!), some of it genetics (I rarely get injured, for whatever reason), some of it just plain luck, like when my knee pain magically went away at mile 13 of the Marine Corps marathon. But let's put aside the idea of doing 52 marathons. Or even running *a* marathon. You don't need to run 26.2 miles...or for that matter, even a half marathon (13.1 miles)...to get the physical and mental benefits of running and physical activity. As your doctor has probably told you, all you need is 30 minutes most days of the week, to make significant improvements in your health.

That's really how I started. And if you're thinking that it might have been easier for me, that's not true. If you're starting this journey from a very low point, a very depressed place, well, sister, I can relate.

As I've related in the pages of this memoir, I began to run out of fear and desperation. I had hit bottom, and my instinct was almost the same as someone in a burning building: Get the hell out of there! Oh yes, I was in bad shape in 2007. I was fat, I was depressed. I was taking too many pills, drinking too much wine, smoking too much weed. My relationships—with my parents, with my kids, with men—were a mess. And on top of it all, I was also spending too much time on my ass, eating too much and feeling sorry for myself.

That's when I started running that day on the beach.

Perhaps you're in a similar place now. Hopefully you're not being called a loser by your dad, or gulping down 100 milligrams of Zoloft a day and washing them down with merlot (which some claim they can do without any problem). Even if you're just someone who'd like to take off a few pounds, and feel better about yourself, getting active will help you in myriad ways. You already know this: Your doctor has probably told you this.

I know something, though, that your doc, your spouse, your boyfriend or girlfriend, might not. I know what it's like to be a woman who is not enamored with her body and her looks, not confident in her abilities, and afraid to take that first step.

If you read psychologist's James Prochaska and Carlo Di Clemente's "stages of change"—a very influential conceptualization on how people adopt new and healthier behaviors (or not)—it is this point, just before taking action, that is the hardest. Prochaska and his colleagues call it "Contemplation," the stage at which you intend to make a change in the near future, but are stuck weighing the pro's and con's. They often become ambivalent; they procrastinate; they become mired in what one researcher described as "chronic contemplation."

If you're reading this, chances are you want to move to that next step, which is Action. But you may have already hamstrung yourself with a bunch of reasons of why you're supposedly not ready. I hear these excuses...and that's what they are...all the time, when it comes to running:

"I don't know what to do once I get out there."

Come on. There are dozens of great and easy-to-follow programs for beginning runners (I asked David to pick three of the best, and they're included at the end of this chapter). Oh, and hello—this is running, not training to write computer code or become a biochemical engineer. It's pretty simple: Step 1: Walk out door. Step 2: Continue walking, briskly but comfortably, for about 20-30 minutes. Congratulations, you've started!

"I have to get the right shoes first."

Hey, I'm always up for shopping. And yes, at some point, you'll want to take a trip to the local running apparel store and find a pair of running shoes that's right for you. But that's no reason to wait. You can get started in whatever you've got. As noted, most beginner running programs have you walking at first, anyway.

"I can't be seen at the gym until I've lost some weight."

You don't have to go to the gym at this point! You can put on your biggest, baggiest sweats, pull a hood up over your head so no one will recognize you, and start walking. No one will even notice you.

Again, excuse, excuses. The biggest obstacle is just getting out the door.

To help you bust out of that contemplation stage and take action — and to offer some practical advice (or laboring under misconceptions) that could save you from making the mistakes I made, here are some ideas to get your inner God or Goddess going:

Running is not sprinting (especially for beginners)

A lot of beginners make the mistake of thinking that if they are going to become runners, they have to run fast. And then when they go out and try to run hard the first time out, they feel miserable, and say they suck at running, and give up.

That's not how you start a running program. Strange as it may sound, you start running by not running: just go out for a brisk walk for 30 minutes. If you choose, you can then gradually build up to a walk/run. Eventually your entire workout is running and even then, it's still usually at a moderate, aerobic pace. Then and only then is it time to think about going faster. If you're a beginner, you're a long way from that now.

Don't make the mistake of thinking that running for health and fitness is an all-out (or as the guys like to say) "balls-to-the-wall" sprint. I'm in awe of the Alison Felix's and Usain Bolt's of the world. But we're not doing what they do.

Do what it takes to make running enjoyable

That moderate, aerobic pace I mentioned in the previous paragraph? Another way that is often described is as a "conversational" pace. Meaning that you can carry on a conversation while you're running. To some, that may come as a surprise. "Talk? Who talks when they run?" *I* do, if I'm running with a group. So do most runners. And most of us who have been involved in the sport for a while have learned how to make it enjoyable.

Run with your dog. (Like I did. I've been running with Jessie for almost 14 years.)

Fine a scenic area to run, like I did. Hawaii might be a bit of a fantasy, but I'm sure there's a nice park or neighborhood nearby.

Listen to your music (although please, be careful. Better on the treadmill than alone, outside, when you can't hear a car coming).

If you're on the treadmill you can also watch your favorite TV show, or listen to your favorite podcast.

Remember also, contrary to the old myth of running as a solitary sport, many runners train today as part of groups, either informal or organized. It was my friends at the L.A. Road Runners who gave me the impetus and support to do my first marathon. We'd run on the Strand—the popular beach path that extends almost 20 miles from Santa Monica south to Torrance Beach. I still run along there with a group at least once a week, as part of my training. It's energizing to feed off of others; it's also how you learn about the sport; and above all, when you're out there engaged in pleasant conversation with a group of like-minded girls (and boys!), you're almost going to forget you are running.

Bottom line: You should do whatever it takes to make it enjoyable. Some runners love this activity from the get-go. Based on my observations, an equal if not greater number don't. But they do find ways to make it tolerable. Run alone, run with a group. Run in the park, run on a treadmill. Regardless, after a few weeks something happens—one day you go out, you run, the at-first-unfamiliar motion feels more natural and fluid, and...presto! It all changes. It's like a sudden and unexpected re-appraisal of that guy in the elevator at work you've seen for months. One morning, you look at him with fresh eyes, and say "hey...he's cute!"

That's often how it is with running. It's not always love at first step, but it's a relationship worth building.

Imagine a fitter, happier you

Body image is a complicated issue. I still struggle with it, like many women. Social media, in my opinion, has intensified it. Go on Facebook and all you see are even more images of beautiful bodies, which in turn magnify our own imperfections. At least in our minds.

And that's where the problem about our bodies usually resides: In our mind. That negative critic; that internal voice telling you that you're fat or ugly. Whether it's cultural, hormonal or just stress-induced, who knows? The key is that we have to try and silence that voice. Remember—most of what that inner critic is telling you is bullshit! You can do anything you put your mind to, you really can. Before you schedule the visit to the cosmetic dermatologist or go for liposuction, listen to me:

This is a better way. Getting out and getting yourself in shape through physical activity is better than some radical, fad diet or surgery (not to mention, less invasive and cheaper!).

When you get out there and take those first steps, *that's* the beginning of your extreme makeover: That's what I was thinking when I was on the beach that day in Hawaii. I thought "This is the start of the new me, the healthy, glowing, happy me, the Julie I want to be."

Am I constantly glowing and deliriously happy, ten years later? Of course not. But I think I look and feel a helluva lot better than I did when I was lying on the couch, feeling sorry for myself. I also have the tools to help me get out of the funks more effectively. One thing I've learned to do is change the conversation... with myself. Instead of constant negative self-talk, I have learned to discern a more positive voice inside my head. Yours is there, too. Just listen! And whenever that inner critic comes creeping in, tell that voice to buzz off. Silence it with it with a more positive affirmation. Just say, "Hey, I'm not going there. Not now, not today."

Instead of going there, go for a run.

Keeping the balls in the air

Research has shown that lack of time is the reason most cited for not starting an exercise program. You really don't need a study to validate that. I hear it from my non-running friends and social media followers all the time. They want to do something good for themselves; they want to walk or run for a charity; they want to make a difference. But they're juggling jobs and family, along with the other emotional constraints we just mentioned.

How do you find time?

Get a little creative. When I'm training for a marathon, I'll often run to work. There's a gym near my office where I'll shower. I leave a change of clothes in my locker. If I could do that, even one day a week, why can't you? Or how about this: Get up a half hour earlier? Just watch a half hour less of TV the night before! Or—an even bigger culprit these days: Carve out time for exercise by spending 30 minutes less a day on social media.

Once you get started, you will be amazed at how good, how empowered, how energized you feel after 30 minutes, even 20 minutes! You'll want to find the time for it. And *then* you will. Because you're not going to want to miss your workout. I refer back to Prochaska's model one more time: The final stage, after contemplation and action is called "maintenance." This is generally after a few months. At this point, the research shows, people are less tempted to relapse; they become more and more confident in their new lifestyle.

That's the ultimate goal: When it becomes a part of your life—a welcome, enjoyable and beneficial part of your life.

Run for a reason

Why should you run? Because of all the benefits that we've discussed and that are well documented in medical literature: For health, for weight control, to offset the effects of too much sitting, for improved mood and self-esteem, running can do that.

You may also decide to run to challenge yourself, to go longer, to go faster. To run the local 10K or to do your first marathon. If performance becomes your goal, great. Races are fun; and they offer the most objective yardstick for measuring progress. It's fun to set goals, it's good for you, and it gives you a sense of purpose. I'll let you in on something: Crossing that marathon finish line every week for a year, I'm told, is like the same feeling you get from heroin. The dopamine and other brain chemicals that the running produced combined with the rush you get from finishing....it was addicting. In a good way.

But I'm here to offer you another reason; the reason that has come to truly define my running.

Do it for a cause. There's really nothing like that. The run then becomes so much bigger than yourself. It might be what it takes to motivate you as well, especially if that cause means something to you.

You can feel good about giving through your running. You can feel good about yourself through your running.

Bottom line: Start running and you'll get healthier. Start running, and you'll feel healthier. Start running, and you'll transform your life. I did it. You can, too. What's stopping you from taking that first step?

Help Us In The Fight Against Pancreatic Cancer

Here are some organizations that are doing great work in the fight against pancreatic cancer, the insidious disease that took my father and then catapulted me on my 52-marathon journey. I have run to raise money for all these charities. Please support these worthy organizations and of course please connect with me at:

www.marathongoddess.com or on Facebook or Instagram

Hirshberg Foundation for Pancreatic Cancer: www.pancreatic.org

Pancreatic Cancer Action Network: www.pancan.org

Project Purple: www.projectpurple.org

Lazarex Cancer Foundation: www.lazarex.org

Dana-Farber Cancer Institute: www.dana-farber.org

Learn about Julie's exciting, new initiative, 52 Races for 52 Faces, and how you can be a part of it. Visit: www.marathongoddess.com

Acknowledgments

First, a special thank you to Rod Chase, The Chase Family and the Fineberg Foundation for their generosity and support in my fight to help raise money to cure pancreatic cancer. And a special thanks to Rod and my colleagues for dealing with me on many a Monday morning, when I dragged myself back to work after flying back from yet another marathon, somewhere.

Debra Englander, your guidance, wisdom and encouragement propelled me into finishing my book proposal.

Kathryn Ford, master life coach, provided guidance, wisdom, feedback and inspiration. You helped make a dream a reality.

Randi Gunther, is more than my clinical psychologist, she has been my spiritual advisor and a source of inspiration. Thank you for your endless support and for always putting me back on track.

Thanks to Mel Robbins for coming into my life at just the right time. Your work has inspired the world. Thank you for inspiring me to get off my ass and get this book done! Keep being awesome!

To the Hirshberg Foundation for Pancreatic Cancer Research, Project Purple, The Pancreatic Cancer Action Network, the Lazerex Foundation, and all those who are on the front lines in search of a cure, thank you. Together we fight and together we will win! Also thanks to all those who allowed me to share their stories on my social media and throughout my 52 marathons. We keep the memories of your loved ones in our heart.

Lupe Romero-De La Cruz, you are my soul sister and my sunshine. A four-time, seven-year pancreatic cancer survivor who amazes us all with her positivity and strength. Lo Tenemos.

Laurence Cohen, Public Relations man par excellence, has been a good friend and a trusted advisor on all things running and fundraising, for many years.

To my friends with the L.A. Road Runners and the L.A. Leggers; and to all those runners, both here in California and around the world, with whom I've shared training miles and marathons—not to mention secrets. Thank you for your endless support and I wish you continued good luck in your running endeavors. We got this!

To the rock star ladies of my running book club, Julie, Gwen, Stephanie A, Stephanie M, Jody, Cristina and Nancy: Love the bond we created, love our runs and love drinking coffee with you after a run to discuss the latest running book.

To John Hanc, my talented editor and co-writer, for his tireless devotion to this project. And to the amazing team of writers, editors and designers that he assembled:

My other co-writer Ali Nolan, Martha Murphy, Kevin Horton, Roshni Ashar and Andrew Hanc. Thank you for helping me create a book that we can all be proud of.

A Message to My Family

To my husband and coach David, for his wisdom, un-relenting patience, guidance and positivity in dealing with my quest. For believing in me, when I didn't believe in myself. For loving me, when I didn't love myself. For reminding me to have fun. Some of the most important moments of my life would not have happened if it weren't for David, including this book. Thanks for always being there. Love you.

To my extremely talented and beautiful sister Diana, thank you for motivating me to go for my dreams. We're two flowers from the same garden, and while it's been a rocky ride, I am grateful for you.

Mom, you gave me life, love, and class. You taught me to shine my own light as bright as I could, and you were always there for me when I was lost and confused. You took care of my children when I couldn't, and you never gave up on me. I know you instilled strength in me and Diana, and you learned that from your parents, Enid and Sam Young. I know my grandfather as the sweetest, most nurturing man in the world, and Nana as a force to be reckoned with. Nana raised millions for Hadassah Hospital in Israel, and she is a great inspiration to me.

Frankie and Samantha, you are the center of my world. You didn't have it easy, and likely felt confused by a mom who was lost and then found. Frankie, my first born, my golden-haired baby, you were the light of your grandfather's eye. You've inherited his talent and his brains. Samantha, while Papa had some harsh words for you, he really loved you--and you showed him. Graduating UCLA with honors and becoming the mother to two beautiful girls, it's clear that you are unstoppable. Michael and Diana, you are my kids now too, a beautiful addition to our family.

To Amelia and Charlotte, my granddaughters, when I look at you, all I see is love. It is a love so pure and I vow to protect it with all my might. Follow your dreams and don't let anyone or anything stand in your way. You are strong, you are powerful, and you are special. You are meant for great things and the world is already better because you are here.

To my first running partner, my dog Jessie. She has been by my side for 16 years. While she can barely walk now, she is still a great motivator and my best friend.

To Frank, my ex-husband for being my friend after everything that's happened. You showed me and our children the importance of family.

Finally, to my Dad, Maurice Weiss. For his hutzpah, charisma, and inspiration. A man who did it his way and showed me how to do it mine. He lived his truth. Thank you, Papa, for your enthusiastic spirit. While I didn't always appreciate it in the past, I sure do now. I wish I could have saved you, I tried. So now I try to save others. When you died, I couldn't let you go, so I found the part of me that is you. In my running, you became my voice. I will continue to use that voice, so we can have a future where no one should ever have to face a diagnosis like yours and can have a fighting chance.

I love each and every one of you.

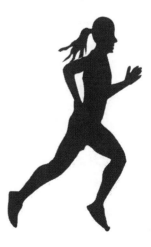

THAT MARATHON YEAR:

Julie Weiss's 52 marathons in 52 weeks

1. 3/18/12 Maritona De Roma   Rome Italy
2. 4/16/12 Boston Marathon   Boston, MA
3. 4/22/12 San Luis Obispo   San Luis Obispo, CA
4. 4/29/12 Big Sur International   Big Sur, CA
5. 5/6/12   Orange County Marathon   Orange County, CA
6. 5/12/12 Grand Valley Marathon   Palisade, CO
7. 5/20/12 Pasadena Marathon   Pasadena, CA
8. 5/27/12 Coeur d'Alene Marathon   Coeur d'Alene, ID
9. 6/3/12   Rock 'n' Roll San Diego   San Diego, CA
10. 6/10/12 Lake Placid Marathon   Lake Placid, NY
11. 6/16/12 Grandma's Marathon   Duluth, MN
12. 6/24/12 Kona Marathon   Kona, HI
13. 6/30/12 Leadville Marathon   Leadville, CO
14. 7/4/12   Foot Traffic Flat Marathon Portland, OR
15. 7/8/12   Missoula Marathon   Missoula, MT
16. 7/15/12 Light at the End of the   Tunnel Issaquah, WA
17. 7/24/12 Deseret Morning News   Salt Lake City, UT
18. 7/29/12 San Francisco Marathon   San Francisco, CA
19. 8/5/12   Extraterrestrial Full Moon Las Vegas, NV
20. 9/2/12   The Kauai Marathon   Kauai, HI
21. 9/9/12   Marathon Madness   Santa Monica, CA
22. 9/16/12 The Maui Marathon   Maui, HI
23. 9/23/12 Half Moon Bay International Half Moon Bay, CA

24. 9/28/12   Emerald Bay Marathon   Lake Tahoe, NV
25. 9/29/12   Cal-Neva Marathon   Lake Tahoe, NV
26. 09/30/12   Lake Tahoe Marathon   Lake Tahoe, NV
27. 10/07/12   Long Beach International   Long Beach, CA
28. 10/14/12   Toronto Waterfront Marathon   Toronto, ON
29. 10/20/12   Hercules: The Journey Begins   Santa Monica, CA
30. 10/21/12   Hercules: The Final Battle   Santa Monica, CA
31. 10/28/12   Marine Corps Marathon   Washington, D.C.
32. 11/04/12   Santa Clarita Marathon   Santa Clarita, CA
33. 11/11/12   Malibu Marathon   Malibu, CA
34. 11/18/12   Route 66 Marathon   Tulsa, OK
35. 11/25/12   Seattle Marathon   Seattle, WA
36. 12/02/12   California International   Sacramento, CA
37. 12/09/12   Honolulu Marathon   Honolulu, HI
38. 12/15/12   Hoover Damn Marathons   Las Vegas, NV
39. 12/22/12   Naughty or Nice   Santa Monica, CA
40. 12/26/12   Operation Jack Marathon   Los Angeles, CA
41. 1/01/13   New Year's Day Marathon   Huntington Beach, CA
42. 1/5/13   Mississippi Blues Marathon   Jackson, MS
43. 1/13/13   Disney World Marathon   Orlando, FL
44. 1/20/13   PF Chang's Rock 'n' Roll   Phoenix, AZ
45. 1/27/13   ING Miami Marathon   Miami, FL
46. 2/3/13   Golden Gate Trail Marathon   Marin County, CA
47. 2/17/13   Surf City Marathon   Huntington Beach, CA
48. 2/17/13   Livestrong Marathon   Austin, TX
49. 2/24/13   New Orleans Rocknroll   New Orleans, LA
50. 3/3/13   Napa Valley Marathon   Napa Valley, CA
51. 3/10/13   Catalina Marathon   Catalina, CA
52. 3/17/13   LA Marathon   Los Angeles, CA

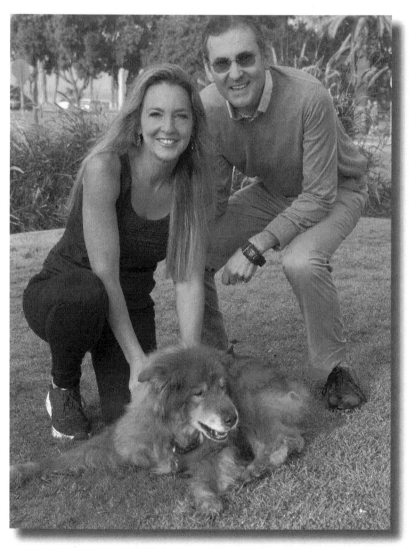

Julie with her husband David and their dog Jessie.

About The Author

Julie Weiss, a/k/a The Marathon Goddess, of Santa Monica, CA., ran 52 marathons in 52 weeks in 2013. In the process, she has raised over $500,000 in the fight against pancreatic cancer through her website:

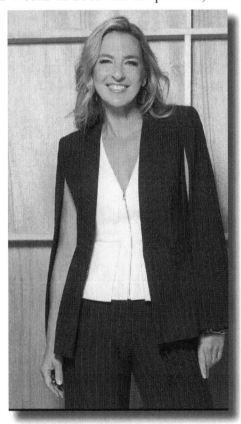

Marathongoddess.com.

Following the death of her father, her biggest fan, from pancreatic cancer, Julie was determined to make a difference. Running marathons gave her the answer. She decided to turn her passion into a purpose and embarked on an almost unprecedented endeavor to raise hope, money and awareness for pancreatic cancer, the third leading cause of cancer death in the United States, and also the lowest funded for research.

Julie has been featured on major media outlets such as CNN, The TODAY Show, the *Los Angeles Times*, *O Magazine* and *Runner's World*. Her story was also told in the inspiring 2012 documentary, *Spirit of the Marathon II*.

Julie, who has now run 105 marathons, chose the name Marathon Goddess, but is quick to point out that its true meaning is not about her; it's a name that allows her to encourage others to embrace their passion and let it shine.

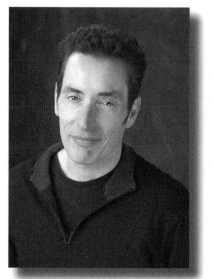
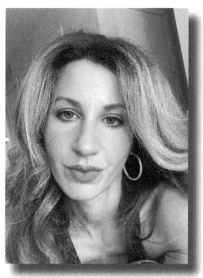

John Hanc has written or co-authored 17 books, including his own award-winning memoir, *The Coolest Race on Earth*, about his experience running the Antarctica Marathon. A long-time contributor to the *New York Times*, *Newsday*, *Smithsonian.com* and *Runner's World*, Hanc teaches journalism at the New York Institute of Technology.

Ali Nolan is a writer and the features editor for *Runner's World* and *Bicycling magazines*. Her byline can also be found in *Sports Literate* and *Garden & Gun*. She holds an MFA from University of North Carolina Wilmington. When not writing or reading, you can find her on the trails.